Review Questions for
NUCLEAR
MEDICINE

The Technology Registry
Examination

Dedicated to my mother
Anna Caiazzo Gallo

and the memory of my father
Ernest Gallo

Review Questions for
NUCLEAR
MEDICINE

The Technology Registry Examination

by

Anna M. Gallo Foss, CNMT, M.B.A.

Medical Imaging Faculty
Springfield Technical Community College

Review Questions Series
Series Editor: Thomas R. Gest, PhD
University of Arkansas for Medical Sciences

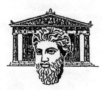

The Parthenon Publishing Group Inc.
International Publishers in Medicine, Science & Technology

One Blue Hill Plaza, Pearl River, New York 10965, USA

Published in the USA by
The Parthenon Publishing Group Inc.
One Blue Hill Plaza,
PO Box 1564, Pearl River,
New York 10965, USA

Published in Europe by
The Parthenon Publishing Group Limited
Casterton Hall, Carnforth,
Lancs LA6 2LA, UK

Library of Congress Cataloging-in-Publication Data

Gallo Foss, Anna M.
    Review questions for nuclear medicine / by Anna M. Gallo Foss.
       p.   cm. – (Review questions series)
    ISBN: 1-85070-703-0
    1. Radioisotope scanning – Examinations, questions, etc. 2. Nuclear medicine –
Examinations, questions, etc. I. Title. II. Series.
    RC78.7.R4G34 1997
    616.07′575′076 – dc21

                                                      96-29859
                                                        CIP

British Library Cataloguing in Publication Data

Gallo Foss, Anna M.
    Review Questions for nuclear medicine
    1. Nuclear medicine – Examinations, questions, etc.
    I. Title
    616′07575′076
    ISBN 1-85070-703-0

This edition published 1997

Printed in the United States

PREFACE

The purpose of almost every review book is to prepare the reader for an imminent exam. This book is no exception. However, in Nuclear Medicine, the technologist who takes the registry exam must know not only about clinical nuclear medicine, but also about physics, chemistry, computers, and radiation safety. Moreover, like everything else in our society, the discipline of nuclear medicine keeps evolving very rapidly. This makes it an interesting specialty, but makes it a bit more challenging for the students and certainly for anyone putting together a review book.

Anna Gallo Foss and her contributors have put together a review book that will satisfy the needs of anyone preparing for the Nuclear Medicine Technology Registry Exam. There is enough of a review of each area to cover the important points. There are then more than enough multiple choice questions on that area to give the student a good sense of what must be known. Finally, a full blown mock registry and some hints on taking a test are included.

It was a pleasure to go through the book, both to see what some of my old students are up to, and to replenish my supply of questions on instrumentation, computers and radiation safety. Although, in my 20 years of teaching the NMT's from this area, I probably have asked most of them already.

Jerome Wagner
Professor of Physics
Rochester Institute of Technology

CONTENTS

Numbers in parentheses indicate number of questions available.

CONTRIBUTORS

Shiela M. Bowler, R.N., M.Ed
Professor, Medical Assisting Program
Springfield Technical Community College
Springfield, MA

David Galleher, RT (R), CNMT
Co-ordinator of Nuclear Medicine Department
Geneva General Hospital
Geneva, NY

Dianne Gilbert, CNMT
Nuclear Medicine Technologist
Harmot Medical Center
Erie, PA

Richard Serino, CNMT, M.Ed.
Department Head, Nuclear Medicine Technology Program
Springfield Technical Community College
Springfield, MA

Scott Surovi, CNMT
Assistant Radiation Safety Officer
Mallinckrodt Medical, INC
Nuclear Medicine Division
Diagnostic Imaging Services
Maryland Heights, MO

Kevin Tracy, CNMT
Manager, Chief Technologist
Gillett Cardiovascular Laboratory
Hartford, CT

Donald C. Tyler, CNMT
Nuclear Medicine Technologist
Harmot Medical Center
Erie, PA

Cheryl Waldman, CNMT
Nuclear Medicine Technologist
Pittsford, NY

INTRODUCTION

A background knowledge and formal instruction in the art and science of nuclear medicine technology is prerequisite to the use of this review book. The review questions may be used concurrently with instruction of concepts and principles. The questions are grouped in topical chapters to assist in identifying gaps in understanding or areas of misinterpretation.

At the beginning of each chapter is a brief summary of content intended to highlight relevant material, rather than provide in-depth instruction. The summaries and questions should be used as an additional study tool in a comprehensive course of study in nuclear medicine technology and in no way as a replacement for formal instruction and clinical practice. The questions are presented in multiple choice format with 2 (true/false) to 5 distracters. Where appropriate, an explanation is provided for the correct answer to help explain the content of the question.

Questions were contributed by allied health faculty and clinical practitioners and every effort has been made to reflect current clinical practice and application. The emphasis is not on recall of basic knowledge, but on the application of that knowledge in clinical practice. Questions that are primarily comprehension are emphasized in the earlier sections of each chapter. I owe a debt of gratitude to the contributors for their fine work and appreciate the clinical expertise that they brought to this review book.

Anna M. Gallo Foss, CNMT, MBA
Professor, Medical Imaging
Springfield Technical Community College

TEST-TAKING TIPS

Before the Examination

Have ready

-admission ticket or admission letter (no candidate will be admitted without the letter or ticket)
-photo identification bearing your signature
 (valid driver's license, passport, student ID)
-if required, a passport-quality photograph
-a map or directions to the test site
-4 or 5 number 2 pencils (sharpened) with erasers
-an accurate watch (not all rooms may have clocks) to help pace yourself
-a basic, nonprogrammable calculator (battery or solar-powered; noiseless). Be sure you are familiar with its use!

Get a good night's sleep. You may want to arrive at the test site city the night before. If not, allow plenty of time to get to the test site on time. (Candidates will not be allowed to take the examination if they arrive late).

Candidates should dress appropriately. Bring a sweater or two; the rooms may be too warm or too cool.

Do not bring books, notes, references, or scrap paper to the examination room. Use your test booklet as scrap paper and write in it. Computerized examinations also allow calculators. Scrap paper will be provided and collected at the end of the examination.

At the Examination

Answer ALL of the questions. Scoring is based on the number of correct answers. There is no penalty for incorrect answers. **On the computerized examinations, you will not be able to skip questions.**

Pace yourself. Don't work so fast that you get careless, but don't spend a lot of time on questions that are too difficult. Use the "best guess" method and fill-in an answer on your answer sheet , mark the question in your test booklet, and return to it at the end, if time permits. **On computerized exams, you will have 15 minutes to learn how to use the system. Pay special attention to explanations on how to "mark" questions you are unsure of so you may go back to specific questions without paging through the entire examination.**

Eliminate as many wrong answers as you can. It is much easier to decide between two answers than five. Make educated guesses.

Read all the answer choices before you decide which one is best.

Don't second guess the question. Make sure you are answering the question being asked and not one that you think is being asked.

When you change an answer, make sure you have a reason for doing so; don't change answers on a last minute "hunch".

On "paper" examinations:
Do not make stray marks on the answer sheet. The examinations are scored by optical scanner and will not discriminate between an accidental mark and a filled-in circle.

Do not fill in more than one answer circle. If you change an answer, erase the incorrect selection completely, and blacken your correct choice.

Check frequently to insure that you are marking your responses in the correct spots; i.e. answer to question number 123 corresponds to number 123 on the answer sheet.

You may use a calculator for solving problems, but not all problems require the use of a calculator and using one can be a time-waster. Don't try to do the calculations in your head. Write in the test booklet.

Have important rules and basic knowledge at your fingertips so that it can be applied to answering questions dealing with job-related tasks.

Review your application booklet for instructions, format, and other tips so you will not waste time at the examination trying to familiarize yourself with the policies and procedures relating to the examination.

SECTION 1: RADIATION HEALTH SAFETY

TUTORIAL

The Nuclear Regulatory Commission (NRC) adopts many of the recommendations and guidelines set by the International Council on Radiation Protection (ICRP) and the National Council on Radiation Protection and Measurement. The *Code of Federal Regulations*, 10CFR20, was revised and were effective as of January 1, 1994. This revision incorporates advances in the science and concepts of radiation protection and principal recommendations of the ICRP.

The principles of radiation protection from external sources are based on the factors of time, distance, shielding, and activity.

The total radiation exposure is directly proportional to the time of exposure to the radiation source. Therefore, to decrease exposure, one should work quickly and efficiently to reduce the amount of time spent near radiation sources.

The intensity of the radiation source varies inversely as the square of the distance from the source to the point of exposure. This principle is more commonly known as the "Inverse Square Law" and can be written,

$$\frac{I1}{I2} = \frac{(D2)^2}{(D1)^2}$$

By doubling the distance, the radiation dose is reduced to one-fourth of the original intensity.

High atomic number (Z) materials can be used to absorb radiation. Lead is used to shield gamma radiation in nuclear medicine departments because of economic reasons. Plastic should be used for radionuclides that emit beta particles (e.g. 32P), because in high Z containers such as lead, they produce highly penetrating bremsstrahlung radiations.

Radiation exposure increases with the intensity of the radioactive materials being used. Whenever possible, avoid working with large amounts of radioactivity or placing yourself in an environment when large amounts are stored.

Film badges and thermoluminescent dosimeters (TLD) are monitoring devices that are commonly used for nuclear medicine personnel. In addition, laboratory coats and gloves should always be worn when working with radioactive materials. Familiarity with receiving and monitoring radioactive packages, radioactive waste disposal, and the records that must be maintained for the receipt, storage, and disposal of radioactive materials is essential.

DIRECTIONS: Each of the numbered items or incomplete statements is followed by answers or by completion of the statement. Select the ONE lettered answer or completion that is BEST in each case.

1.001 The three most important factors to be considered when handling radioactive materials are:
   A. activity, distance, type of emission
   B. organ sensitivity, type of emission, distance
   C. type of emission, shielding, area of exposure
   D. time of exposure, distance, shielding

D. is correct.
Minimizing the amount of time spent in a radioactive area, increasing the distance from a radiation source, and using a shielding material such as lead, are three practical methods for reducing exposure from radiation.

1.002 The ALARA concept in radiation protection refers to:
   A. as long as radiation is around
   B. personnel can accumulate up to the maximum amount permitted
   C. personnel should be notified by the radiation safety officer if radiation exposure exceeds the maximum permitted
   D. keeping personnel exposure to radiation as low as reasonably achievable

D. is correct.
ALARA stands for "As Low As Reasonably Achievable" which is a philosophy to increase awareness and reduce radiation exposure incorporating reasonable cost in effort to reduce exposure.

1.003 If the intensity of radiation is 10 mrem/hour at 2 meters from the source, the intensity at 8 meters from the source is _____ mrem/hour.
   A. 0.625
   B. 2.5
   C. 40
   D. 160

A. is correct.
The Inverse Square Law is expressed as:

$$\frac{I_1}{I_2} = \frac{(D_2)^2}{(D_1)^2} \qquad \text{therefore,} \qquad \frac{10}{X} = \frac{(8)^2}{(2)^2}$$

$$40 = 64X; \ X = 0.625$$

1.004 Upon arrival, a package containing radioactive material with a DOT Category II yellow label must have a dose rate which at the surface does not exceed:
   A. .5 mrem/hour
   B. 5 mrem/hour
   C. 25 mrem/hour
   D. 50 mrem/hour

D. is correct.
The Department of Transportation controls the packaging and transportation of materials containing radioactivity. A category II yellow label is less than or equal to 50 mrem/hr at the surface of the package and less than or equal to 1 mrem/hr measured at 1 meter distance.

1.005 If you work in an area where a major part of your body could receive greater than 5 mrem in any one hour or more than 100 mrem in five consecutive days, the sign posted would be:
   A. Caution: Radiation Materials
   B. Caution: Radiation Area
   C. Caution: High Radiation Area
   D. no signage is necessary

B. is correct.
Nuclear Regulatory Commission (NRC), Title 10, Code of Federal Regulations

1.006 Personnel radiation exposure records should be kept:
   A. indefinitely
   B. 2 years
   C. 3 years
   D. 5 years

A. is correct.
Personnel radiation exposure records should be kept indefinitely.

1.007 Aspects of radioactive materials which are under strict federal regulations include all of the following EXCEPT:
- A. production
- B. price
- C. possession
- D. use
- E. disposal

B. is correct.
Rules regarding the production, use, and disposal of radioactive materials and supporting documentation must be adhered to.

1.008 The best way for a technologist to decontaminate a ^{99m}Tc pertechnatate spill to the hands is by the use of:
- A. decay
- B. alcohol
- C. soap and water
- D. an alkaline cleanser

C. is correct.
Avoid hot water and strong soaps; a mild soap and warm water should be used to clean the skin.

1.009 If a misadministration of a patient dose occurs and is documented on March 3, 1996, the earliest date that those records may be destroyed is:
- A. after March 3, 1999
- B. after March 3, 2001
- C. after March 3, 2003
- D. after March 3, 2006

D. is correct.
Misadministration records must be kept for ten years.

1.010 Radioactive materials that decayed through ten physical half-lives are reduced to:
- A. background
- B. less than 5 mrem/hr
- C. less than 2 mrem/hr
- D. less than .2mrem/hr

A. is correct.
After ten physical half-lives, a radioactive material is reduced to background levels.

1.011 The intensity of radiation is 100 mrem/hr at a distance of 9 feet from the source. The intensity at 3 feet from the source is _____ mrem/hour.
- A. 33.3
- B. 300
- C. 333
- D. 900

D. is correct.
The Inverse Square Law is expressed as:

$$\frac{I1}{I2} = \frac{(D2)^2}{(D1)^2} \qquad \text{therefore,} \qquad \frac{100}{X} = \frac{(3)^2}{(9)^2}$$

$$8100 = 9X; \text{ so } X = 900$$

1.012 When a radiation worker will be exposed to large amounts of radiation are on an infrequent schedule, the monitoring device(s) which would be most useful is(are):
- A. thermoluminescent dosimeters (TLD)
- B. film badge and ring (TLD) badge
- C. pocket dosimeter and TLD
- D. A and B

C. is correct.
Pocket dosimeters (ionization chambers) are useful as supplementary monitoring devices giving an immediate read-out of radiation exposure. The TLD will give an exposure reading over a period of time and is a permanent record of the worker's exposure.

1.013 What is the easiest and most practical way for a technologist to reduce the radiation exposure from patients injected for nuclear medicine studies?
- A. lead shielding and lead aprons
- B. distance
- C. limitation of time of exposure
- D. concrete shielding

B. is correct.
Increasing the distance from the source of radiation (the patient) is the most practical way to decrease the amount of radiation received without compromising patient care or the quality of the study.

1.014 A radiation beam of 100 mrem/hr is reduced to 25 mrem/hr by an attenuating material. This material is equal to _____ half value layers (HVL).
   A. 2
   B. 3
   C. 4
   D. 5
   E. none of the above

E. is correct.
One HVL reduces the radiation intensity to half its original value. One HVL reduces 100 mrem/hr to 50 mrem/hr; another HVL reduces the 50 mrem/hr by one-half again or to 25 mrem/hr.

1.015 The most important factor(s) in reducing the radiation dose to the patient include:
   A. the correct radiopharmaceutical and dose is administered to the patient
   B. the dose calibrator is calibrated to ensure accurate readings
   C. the imaging equipment is checked to ensure proper function
   D. all of the above
   E. both A and B

E. is correct.
The correct dose and assay are critical in limiting exposure to the patient and are in keeping with the ALARA principle. Imaging equipment should be checked before patients are injected for a study and dose not contribute directly to the radiation dose to the patient.

1.016 A technologist must use syringe shields while administering a dose to the patient, but may prepare radiopharmaceuticals without a syringe shield as long as there are no other individuals in the radiopharmacy during the preparation.
   A. true
   B. false

B. is correct.
Syringe shields are required both during radiopharmaceutical kit preparation and administration of dose to a patient.

1.017 The first person a staff technologist should report an excessive radiation exposure to is:
   A. the nuclear medicine physician
   B. the RSO (Radiation Safety Officer)
   C. the NRC (Nuclear Regulatory Commission)
   D. the chief technologist
   E. B or D

E. is correct.
The chief technologist or RSO (in some departments this is the same person), are responsible for the implementation of regulations regarding radiation exposure. This person will follow the proper procedure for notification of incidents.

1.018 The dose for a radionuclide gated blood pool study in your facility is 20 mCi of ^{99m}Tc pertechnatate. A patient is given a dose of 5 mCi of ^{99m}Tc pertechnatate intravenously and a diagnostic study performed. The dose was:
   A. a misadministration, the dose was more than 50% different from the prescribed dose
   B. incorrectly administered by intravenous injection
   C. correctly administered, as long as a diagnostic study is achieved
   D. A and B

A. is correct.
According to the NRC, the dose was a misadministration since it differed from the prescribed dose by more than 50%.

1.019 While adhering to the ALARA principle is important for radiation workers, it is not a concern for the patient since the benefit of the study outweighs the risks of radiation exposure.
   A. true
   B. false

B. is correct.
While a study may be of benefit to a patient, adherence to ALARA principles and "doing it right the first time" will ensure that exposure is kept as low as reasonably achievable.

1.020 Urine from a Schilling's test must be kept in storage for a period of ten half-lives before it can be disposed of into the sanitary sewer.
  A. true
  B. false

B. is correct.
Urine, stool, and vomitus from a patient may be discarded into the sanitary sewer.

1.021 Before a package that transported a radioactive material can be discarded, you should:
  A. store for a period of ten days
  B. store for a period of ten half-lives
  C. flatten the cardboard to facilitate disposal
  D. deface the radioactive transport label
  E. none of the above

D. is correct.
As long as the package is uncontaminated, defacing or removing the label is all that is required.

1.022 A package arrives with a half-life of 8 days and a total quantity of 30 mCi. According to the NRC regulations:
  A. a wipe test is necessary
  B. the package is exempt from wipe test requirements
  C. the NRC should be notified immediately
  D. the package should be returned to the carrier

B. is correct.
Packages with a half-life of less than 30 days and a total amount of radioactivity less than 100 MCi do not require a wipe test on the external package surface.

1.023 The dose limit for members of the public includes both external and internal doses.
  A. true
  B. false

A. is correct.
The dose limit of public individual is 500 mrem/year from all sources excluding natural background and medical diagnostic and therapeutic doses.

1.024 A 20 mCi dose of ^{99m}Tc HDP results in a total body absorbed dose of approximately 0.25 rads. This value is equivalent to:
  A. 0.25 rem
  B. 2.50 mGy
  C. 0.50 mSv
  D. 0.25 Gy

B. is correct.
Absorbed dose =
.25 rads x $\frac{1 Gy}{100 rad}$ = .0025 Gy = .25 cGy = 2.5 mGy

1.025 Of the following sources used to calibrate a dose calibrator, which has the longest half-life?
  A. 133 Ba
  B. 137 Cs
  C. ^{99m}Tc
  D. 57 Co

B. is correct.
T1/2 137 Cs = 30.17 years;
T1/2 133 Ba = 10.66 years;
T1/2 57 Co = 270 days;
T1/2 ^{99m}Tc = 6 hours

1.026 The ^{99}Mo column, if separated from a ^{99}Mo/^{99m}Tc generator, must be held for at least _____ prior to disposal as nonradioactive waste.
  A. 60.2 hours
  B. 10 days
  C. 660 hours
  D. 30 days

C. is correct.
The half-life of ^{99}Mo is 66 hours. It is recommended to store a material for a minimum of 10 half-lives and then carefully monitor for decay to background before disposal in the regular trash. Thus, 660 hours would be the minimum amount of time for ^{99}Mo to decay-in-storage.

1.027 A 10 mCi dose of a radionuclide would be equal to what activity in becquerels?
  A. 3.7 Bq
  B. 37 Bq
  C. 370 Bq
  D. 37 MBq
  E. 370 MBq

E. is correct.
Activity in Bq
 = 10 mCi x $(10^{-3} \frac{Ci}{mCi})$ x $(3.7 \times 10^{10} \frac{Bq}{Ci})$
 = 10 x 10^{-3} x 3.7 x 10^{10} Bq
 = 3.7 x 10^8 Bq   = 370 x 10^6 Bq
          = 370 MBq

1.028 A dose equivalent of 20 mSv is equal to:
   A. 1 mrem
   B. 2 mrem
   C. 1 rem
   D. 2 rem

D. is correct.
In traditional units the dose equivalent is the rem. One (1) Sv = 100 rem; so 20 mSv = 2 rem. The dose equivalent in sievert (Sv) is equal to the absorbed dose in gray (Gy), traditionally rad, multiplied by the appropriate quality factor.

1.029 Venting of 133Xe gas to the atmosphere is acceptable in all of the conditions EXCEPT:
   A. a rooftop designated as a restricted area
   B. an activated charcoal filter is used as a trap
   C. the activity released is 10% or less of legal requirements
   D. all of above

D. is correct.
All are acceptable conditions to reduce the amount of activity released to the atmosphere.

1.030 Proper technique in administering a radiopharmaceutical includes:
   A. use of syringe shields
   B. use of disposable gloves
   C. recapping syringe needles that have been in contact with patients
   D. all of above
   E. A and B only

E. is correct.
Unless their use interferes with, or prevents the efficient accomplishment of the injection, syringe shield and disposable gloves should be used in both preparation and administration of all radiopharmaceuticals. OSHA (Occupational Safety and Health Administration) requires that workers NOT recap syringe needles used for patients.

1.031 Factors that should be considered by the technologist in an effort to apply the ALARA principle to patients include:
   A. administration of the correct dose of radiopharmaceutical to the patient
   B. proper calibration of the dose calibrator to ensure its accurate performance
   C. appropriate quality assurance tests on imaging equipment to ensure proper function
   D. all of the above
   E. both A and B

D. is correct.
The imaging equipment does not directly affect the amount of radiation that a patient is exposed to. However, if the scintillation camera is not functioning properly and the patient must return for a repeat study, and an additional dose, it would certainly be within the technologists responsibility in insuring the principles of ALARA are upheld.

SECTION 2: NUCLEAR MEDICINE TECHNOLOGY INSTRUMENTATION

TUTORIAL

There are instruments and equipment used in nuclear medicine that would be considered the "work-horses" of the department. It is the basic equipment that this chapter deals with; those instruments that are common to every nuclear medicine department and whose quality control tests are familiar to every nuclear medicine technologist.

The simplest of the gas-filled detectors is the ionization chamber. If a source of radioactivity is placed in an ionization chamber, an electrical current will be generated that is directly proportional to the quantity of radioactivity in the chamber. The ionization current is also affected by the energy of the radionuclide. As a result, a milliCurie of one radionuclide will not generate the same current as a milliCurie of another radionuclide. This is the basic principle of operation of a dose calibrator. The dose calibrator should be calibrated for every radionuclide to be assayed. Constancy should be checked daily with a long-lived source of known activity.

The Geiger-Muller (GM), or Geiger counter is another example of a gas-filled detector. Their use in nuclear medicine laboratories is primarily to monitor or survey for possible contamination of personnel, work spaces, or packages. Daily reference checks using constant geometry should be performed to verify calibration of the survey instrument.

The gamma scintillation spectrometer allows the user to discriminate different gamma energies, i.e., to analyze the gamma energies that are detected by the scintillation crystal. Scintillation cameras and well counters are able to perform gamma energy selection. One of the major features of the scintillation detection system is that the output signal is proportional to the energy deposited in the crystal. This allows selection of pulses that are to be accepted for processing.

The gamma scintillation camera consists of a collimator, crystal (usually NaI (Tl), photomultiplier tubes, and electronics to sort out and localize the signal for display. Collimators limit the entry of gamma rays that can interact with the crystal so that the point of origin of the scintillation event can be localized. The gamma ray entering through the collimator, interacts in the crystal producing a portion of energy in the form of light to viewed by the photomultiplier tubes.

Uniformity of a scintillation camera refers to the response of the camera to a uniform field of radiation (or flood source). There should be a daily check made by visual or computer inspection of the flood image. Spatial resolution tests the scintillation camera system's ability to accurately reproduce small differences in the concentration of radionuclides in closely spaced areas.

The performance of the scintillation system should be checked daily to insure the acquisition of diagnostic images. Changes in electrical power supply, physical shock, temperature changes, humidity, dust, background radiation, and radiofrequency interference can affect the performance of the imaging system. Sources that are close in energy to the most commonly used radiopharmaceuticals should be used for quality control testing.

An important measurement to assess the efficiency of the scintillation counting equipment in a nuclear medicine department is the full width at half maximum (FWHM), which should typically be less than 10%. The formula for determining the percent energy resolution for a particular radionuclide is:

$$\% \text{ energy resolution} = \frac{\text{FWHM}}{\text{photopeak}} \times 100$$

2.001 The amount of light generated by a sodium iodide crystal is directly related to the:
   A. photon energy absorbed in the crystal
   B. diameter of the crystal
   C. thickness of the crystal
   D. age of the crystal

A. is correct.
A NaI (Tl) scintillation detector provides an output signal from the photomultiplier tube that is proportional in amplitude to the amount of energy absorbed in the crystal.

2.002 The photo peak of a spectrum of ^{99m}Tc represents gamma rays which:
   A. interact only by photoelectric effect
   B. interact in the crystal and deposit all of their energy there
   C. interact only by Compton scatter
   D. none of the above

B. is correct.
Most photoelectric interactions result in full deposition of the gamma energy in the detector.

2.003 If the FWHM Full Width Half Maximum) is 15 keV, what is the energy resolution for a peak of ^{99m}Tc?
   A. 2%
   B. 7.5%
   C. 11 %
   D. 15%

C. is correct.
% energy resolution is equal to the FWHM divided by the peak energy (140 keV) times 100.
($\underline{15}$ x 100 = 11%)
   140

2.004 Of the following, the two most important quality assurance measurements of a scintillation camera imaging system are:
   A. focus; astigmatism
   B. energy resolution; counting efficiency
   C. field uniformity; spatial resolution
   D. dead time; resolving time

C. is correct.
Spatial resolution is a determinant of image quality, while field uniformity assesses detector performance.

2.005 Which of the following radionuclides would be used as a source to calibrate a detection system used for ^{99m}Tc?
   A. Cs 137
   B. Cr 51
   C. Co 57
   D. Ba 133

C. is correct.
Co 57
The energy of 57Co (122 keV) is closest to ^{99}mTc (140 keV).

2.006 The basic function of all collimators is to:
   A. increase the resolution of the instruments
   B. increase the efficiency of the instruments
   C. limit scattered radiation
   D. limit access of photons to the instrument

D. is correct.
Absorptive collimation allows only a fraction of the gamma rays striking the collimator to actually pass through onto the detector.

2.007 For a parallel hole collimator, the best resolution is at:
   A. the focal distance
   B. the collimator surface
   C. 5 cm
   D. 15 cm

B. is correct.
Resolution is always best with the source of activity as close to the collimator as possible.

2.008 When one increases the resolution of a collimator, its efficiency:
   A. increases
   B. decreases
   C. remains the same

B. is correct.
For a given septal thickness, collimator resolution increases (or is improved) at the cost of decreased efficiency as photon discrimination increases.

2.009 The resolving power of collimators decreases with increasing gamma ray energy because of:
   A. increased Compton scatter
   B. increased geometric losses
   C. increased septal penetration
   D. decreased stopping power

C. is correct.
If collimator septa are too thin, higher energy gamma rays will penetrate to the detector resulting in loss of image contrast and spatial resolution.

2.010 Of the following choices, which collimator is used for thyroid uptake studies with radio iodine?
   A. flat field
   B. diverging
   C. converging
   D. pinhole
   E. medium energy

A. is correct.
Flat field collimators in the uptake probe are used because of their high efficiency and uniform response field.

For the following three questions, assume you are working with a scintillation counter with a normal gain switch, with gains of 4, 8, and 16. The SCA has a baseline which adjusts from 1 - 1000 and a differential window that also adjusts from 0 to 1000. The unit is calibrated with the gain set at 8, so that each division on the SCA is equal to 1 keV.

2.011 In order to count the 320 keV peak of Cr-51 with a 15% window the window should be set at _____ keV.
   A. 15
   B. 24
   C. 30
   D. 48

D. is correct.
15% of 320 keV is 48 keV (320 x .15 = 48)

2.012 For a 15% window (photo peak 320), the baseline of the SCA should be set at:
   A. 296
   B. 305
   C. 320
   D. 368

A. is correct.
320 - 24 = 296 (24 keV is one half of the window)

2.013 With the gain set at 4, the baseline at 785, and the window at 50 keV; what is the energy of the photo peak found in the center of the window?
   A. 785 keV
   B. 810 keV
   C. 1570 keV
   D. 1595 keV

D. is correct.
Since the unit was calibrated with the gain set at 8, the energy would be twice what is read on the scale.
With true gain, when the gain is halved, the energy range is increased. (785 x 2 = 1570 + 25 keV = 1595 keV)

2.014 All of the following are gas detectors EXCEPT:
   A. gamma scintillation camera
   B. "cutie-pie" survey meter
   C. dose calibrator
   D. Geiger-Mueller counter

A. is correct.
A gamma camera is a scintillation counter.

2.015 Dose calibrators are examples of a(n):
   A. ionization chamber
   B. solid scintillation system
   C. liquid scintillation system
   D. Geiger-Mueller detector

A. is correct.
A dose calibrator is a gas ionization chamber.

2.016 If a noticeable change in field uniformity of a gamma scintillation camera occurs, the technologist should first check the:
  A. temperature
  B. photo peaking
  C. collimator
  D. system for contamination

B. is correct.
A common cause of nonuniformity is a misadjusted photo peak. Since it is also easily resolved, it should be checked first when the flood field image is noticeably different from day to day.

2.017 Of the following phantoms to assess spatial resolution, the only one that determines the resolution of all areas of the detector with one image is the _____ phantom.
  A. Hine-Duley
  B. four-quadrant
  C. parallel-line equal-space (PLES)
  D. orthogonal hole

D. is correct.
The orthogonal hole phantom consists of holes of equal diameter at right angles to each other that cover the entire surface of the detector.

2.018 In addition to spatial resolution, what other parameter of the detection system can be assessed with either a bar or orthogonal hole phantom?
  A. sensitivity
  B. uniformity
  C. spatial linearity
  D. geometric variation

C. is correct.
Spatial linearity can be assessed by evaluating the "straightness" of parallel bars or parallel rows of holes.

2.019 One of the advantages of the "cutie pie" as a survey meter is that it:
  A. responds only to contamination levels of radiation
  B. is independent of the energy of the radiation
  C. responds only to high level radiation
  D. responds only to low level radiation

B. is correct.
The "Cutie Pie" survey meter gives a true value regardless of the type of energy of radiation.

2.020 The primary difference between the Cutie Pie detector and a Geiger Mueller detector is:
  A. method of detection
  B. operating potential
  C. display modes
  D. ambient potential

B. is correct.
The two types of survey meters are the "Cutie Pie" which is an ionization type and the Geiger-Mueller (G-M) type.

2.021 Of the following dose calibrator quality control tests, which is required to be tested daily by the NRC?
  A. geometric dependence
  B. activity linearity
  C. constancy
  D. accuracy

C. is correct.
Constancy, or the ability of the dose calibrator to reproduce measurements of a source of known activity from day to day is required to be tested daily and be within 10% of the decay corrected activity of the standard sample.

2.022 When assaying a patient dose, if the sample is elevated slightly in the dose calibrator, the dose read-out will be _____ .
  A. higher than the actual dose
  B. lower than the actual dose
  C. the same as the actual dose

B. is correct.
Geometry and volume can affect the measurement of a patient dose. Syringe size, dose concentration, and containers (vial vs syringe) can affect the reading from the true or actual activity of the source.

2.023 When performing quality control tests of constancy, accuracy, linearity, and geometric variation, the NRC directs correction by repair, replacement, or use of correction factors, if the error is greater than:
   A. 5%
   B. 10%
   C. 15 %
   D. 20%

B. is correct.
Errors greater than 10% of actual activity readings require corrective action. In addition, the NRC requires that quality control records be retained for 3 years.

2.024 Percent energy resolution is defined or calculated as follows:
   A. photo peak energy (keV) / FWHM (keV)
   B. photo peak energy (keV) / FWHM (keV) X 100
   C. FWHM (keV) / photo peak energy (keV)
   D. FWHM (keV) / photo peak energy (keV) X 100

D. is correct.
In the ideal, a pulse height spectra would have sharp lines and edges, with one single line representing the photo peak. With NaI detectors, we see a range of energies and the photo peak is a Poisson or Gaussian shaped curve. The width of this curve, measured across half the amplitude (FWHM) is the energy resolution, most often expressed as a percent of the photo peak.

2.025 Reasons why good energy resolution is a desirable characteristic for a NaI detector include:
   A. precise identification of gamma rays
   B. separation of gamma energies that are similar
   C. reduces number of photoelectrons released per keV
   D. all of the above
   E. A and B only

E. is correct.
For radionuclide identification and scatter reduction, good energy resolution allows greater precision. A reduction in the number of photoelectrons released per keV will cause a degradation in energy resolution.

2.026 Energy resolution of a NaI detecting system increases with increasing gamma ray energy. Expressed as %FWHM, this means that the %FWHM _____ as gamma energy increases.
   A. increases
   B. decreases
   C. remains the same

B. is correct.
The %FWHM becomes smaller or decreases with increasing gamma ray energies and the % statistical variation decreases. Lower %FWHM indicates a system with better resolution than a system with a higher %FWHM.

2.027 Counting errors above those that could be predicted using Poisson statistics can be checked for using the _____ test.
   A. linearity
   B. Chi-Square
   C. reference check
   D. energy resolution

B. is correct.
Random counting errors that are greater than those predicted may be encountered in nuclear medicine instruments because of malfunctions of the equipment. Random errors which are variations in results from one measurement to the next, result from the nature of radioactive decay. The chi-square test will check for those errors greater than predicted, indicating malfunction rather than random decay.

2.028 The nuclear medicine technologist performs a chi-square test and finds a p value that is 0.5. This would indicate that:
   A. the instrument is counting within an acceptable range and variations match the expected
   B. the range is unacceptable and variations do not match the expected
   C. the instrument should not be used until replaced or repaired
   D. the test is equivocal and should be repeated
   E. none of the above

A. is correct.
Acceptable p values lie between 0.1 and 0.9. Values that lie outside that range indicate that the variations are not within the predicted range for random decay variations.

2.029 A uniform response to a wide range of radioactivities is a parameter of dose calibrator performance known as:
   A. accuracy
   B. precision
   C. linearity
   D. geometric calibration

2.030 The parameter that measures the degree to which a dose calibrator measures sample or patient doses that agree with actual or true doses is:
   A. accuracy
   B. precision
   C. linearity
   D. geometric calibration

2.031 The sensitivity of the dose calibrator chamber to different source configurations is measured by:
   A. accuracy
   B. precision
   C. linearity
   D. geometric calibration

2.032 The ability of the dose calibrator to consistently reproduce results of activity measurements is:
   A. accuracy
   B. precision
   C. linearity
   D. geometric calibration

C. is correct.
Linearity of a dose calibrator measures response at different activity levels. The dose calibrator should function linearly (with accuracy) from the highest dose that will be administered to a patient to 10 uCi of activity.

A. is correct.
If activity measurements of a standard source fall within 10% of the calculated activity for that standard, the instrument is functioning with acceptable accuracy.

D. is correct.
Changing the vial or syringe size or sample volume can significantly affect the measurement of activity and correction factors should be established for significant changes that would affect dose activity readings.

B. is correct.
Precision or constancy is checked daily to insure that the instrument consistently reads activity over the range of frequently used radionuclides.

SECTION 3: COMPUTERS IN NUCLEAR MEDICINE

TUTORIAL

The use of computers can be applied to nearly every study that is performed in nuclear medicine whether as a "back-up" to planar acquisition of images, or as a necessity to acquisition and processing as in nuclear cardiology and SPECT reconstruction. The ability to quantify and manipulate information mathematically has increased the sensitivity and utility of many studies that are performed in nuclear medicine today.

Clinical studies can be greatly affected by the flexibility provided by the software for data acquisition, post-processing of data, user-friendliness, and presentation of images for display and evaluation. Artifacts that are introduced because of poor quality control techniques can grossly affect the final results leading to misdiagnosis or an increase in repeat studies.

In nuclear medicine we are looking at the basic interface between the gamma scintillation camera and the computer to acquire, process, and display count information available from the "sample" or patient. Analog scintillation cameras which produce a signal in which voltage changes with time require an analog-to-digital converter (ADC) to convert the analog signal to the digital signal needed by the computer. With advances in microprocessor technology, digital scintillation cameras are now available increasing the speed of acquisition, data storage, and display.

The computer can be used for nonuniformity correction, background correction and smoothing, zoom mode acquisition, attenuation correction, as well as numerous acquisition techniques that take advantage of the speed and mathematical positioning of signals that allows post-processing of information.

It is also important that the technologist be aware of environmental concerns when working with computers. Cleanliness and a relatively dust-free environment should clearly be a priority in any department. Temperature and humidity are factors that should also be of concern; high temperatures can damage the electronic components and low humidity can result in static which can damage computer components and cause loss of data on storage disks. Temperatures should be in the range of 68 - 72 degrees F, with a relative humidity of approximately 40 - 50%.

For the technologist in a modern nuclear medicine department, knowledge of the functions and capabilities of the computer is a vital component in delivering quality, diagnostic images for interpretation by the nuclear medicine physician. The hardware (CPU, memory, input/output devices, data storage), software (operating system, acquisition programs, image processing, SPECT imaging), and the clinical applications of a particular imaging department, should be familiar to all nuclear medicine technologists and physicians in that department to insure efficient and appropriate application of the technology.

3.001 All SPECT imaging devices are computer controlled for both data acquisition and data analysis.
   A. true
   B. false

A. is correct.
The computer has made SPECT imaging possible in both coordinating the collection of data and in performing the complex calculations necessary for reconstruction in image production and analysis.

3.002 Pixels are picture elements of the image matrix that represent individual location counts in the x and y directions. In SPECT imaging, adding depth makes pixels become:
   A. matrices
   B. point sources
   C. vertical elements
   D. volume elements

D. is correct.
Volume elements, or voxels, represent the pixel with the added dimension of depth, or volume.

3.003 In SPECT imaging, parallel-hole collimators are used to insure that the detectors see only the photons along a narrow band that extends from the detector to organ in the radius of rotation. This narrow band is called a:
   A. column
   B. ray
   C. fan
   D. beam

B. is correct.
A composite of the ray sums is the basis for back projection reconstruction. It may be defined as an even projection along the path of the acquired angle.

3.004 Scanning of a ray across a plane in the subject at a particular angular increment forms a(n):
   A. projection
   B. plane
   C. funnel
   D. column

A. is correct.
The number of projection images will vary with the size of the object being imaged and the resolution of the camera system. A projection is simply the count rate profile of the subject at a specified angular orientation.

3.005 After a complete set of projections are obtained, the computer sorts the data and reconstructs an image of the activity distribution in the _____ of interest.
   A. projection
   B. plane
   C. funnel
   D. column

B. is correct.
Using a backprojected image which represents a composite of all the ray sums in a cross-sectional view of the original field, the image is reconstructed.

3.006 The "star" effect in image reconstruction may be created by:
   A. septal penetration
   B. patient motion
   C. collimator contamination
   D. artifacts produced by the overlapping of ray sums
   E. all of the above

D. is correct.
"Star" artifacts are not present in the original object and will degrade images and decrease resolution.

3.007 The "star" effect may be reduced by:
   A. increasing the acquisition time per angle
   B. increasing the count rate
   C. increasing the number of projections acquired
   D. increasing the target-to-detector distance

C. is correct.
Increasing the number of projections acquired can significantly reduce the "star" effect. Note that there is no increase in collection time and sufficient counts per pixel should be provided in a high count study.

3.008 The "star" artifact may be removed by:
   A. back projection
   B. filtering
   C. using only point sources
   D. increasing detector-source distance

B. is correct.
The introduction of a filter to individual projections is one of the most common methods for removing the "star" artifact.

3.009 Attenuation correction methods are used in SPECT imaging because:
   A. most SPECT studies are high-count studies which need to be averaged
   B. attenuation is NOT a problem with SPECT imaging
   C. the attenuation of photons by the patient's body makes it difficult to obtain accurate radiotracer uptake information
   D. areas of increased activity will be demonstrated that are not representative of the subject uptake

C. is correct.
Photons that originate in the center of the subject are more likely to be absorbed (attenuated) by overlying structures than those at the periphery of the subject. Manufacturers have software correcting for attenuation loses.

3.010 Accurate quantitative information about radiopharmaceutical uptake in SPECT imaging is limited by:
   A. patient motion
   B. limited patient dose
   C. high count rates
   D. attenuation of photons by the patient's body

D. is correct.
The definition of attenuation is the absorption of a photon, or charged particle, by matter. The attenuation by the patient's body will affect the quantification of radiopharmaceutical distribution.

3.011 The center of rotation analysis correction program:
   A. should be applied with each collimator change
   B. interprets the axis of rotation for each patient
   C. compensates for minor misalignments
   D. all of above
   E. A and C

E. is correct.
Center of rotation can correct slight misalignments of the imaging system for each projection's interpretation of the camera's axis of rotation. A collimator shift during the detector's rotational path can affect x, y placement of the digital image.

3.012 One of the most prevalent causes of defects seen in the reconstructed SPECT image is the result of:
   A. improper data entry by the technologist
   B. patient motion
   C. gamma camera non-uniformity
   D. collimator misalignment

C. is correct.
A small difference in field uniformity may create numerous artifacts in the reconstructed image. Uniformity correction is one of the most important quality control procedures associated with SPECT imaging.

3.013 A circular path of a "cold" area and ring and "bull's-eye" artifacts are the result of:
   A. improper data entry by the technologist
   B. patient motion
   C. gamma camera non-uniformity
   D. collimator misalignment

C. is correct.
The "bull's-eye" artifact is a summation of an area of decreased activity caused by a field non-uniformity. It is a circular artifact that represents the same geometric configuration as the detector rotation.

3.014 Although manufacturers may differ on uniformity correction flood techniques, the one recommendation by all vendors is:
   A. use of a large, 57Co flood source
   B. monthly acquisition of a correction flood
   C. use of a high count flood correction matrix
   D. use of refillable flood sources for 67Ga, 111In, and 123I

C. is correct.
Correction floods with high counting statistics will lessen the influence of field non-uniformities. A 30 million count flood would yield an expected standard deviation of 1% with lower amplification of artifacts in the reconstructed images.

3.015 Including an area of the patient with an infiltrated dose in the field of view will result in an artifact called:
  A. "bulls-eye"
  B. edge artifact
  C. matrix overflow
  D. star artifact

D. is correct.
Unwanted "hot" spots that are not on the area of interest but included in the field of view will create "star" artifacts that cross on the target organ.

3.016 An increase in matrix size from 64 x 64 byte mode to 128 x 128 word mode for SPECT imaging will result in a _____ factor increase in time and computer storage space.
  A. 2
  B. 4
  C. 8
  D. 16
  E. 32

B. is correct.
In addition to all aspects of the study being increased by a factor of 4, the counts per pixel will be reduced by a factor of 4 reducing the statistical significance of the study.

3.017 When a technologist is setting up for a SPECT acquisition, selection of the acquisition time should include consideration of:
  A. the computer memory available
  B. the speed of the processing program
  C. the patient's ability to hold still
  D. the resolution required for the study
  E. A and C only
  F. C and D only

F. is correct.
A successful study requires that the patient remain still for the duration of the study and a realistic evaluation of the patient's physical and mental status should be made. The technologist must select those imaging parameters that fit both the needs of the patient and the requirements of the study.

3.018 The filter algorithm selected by the technologist should include consideration of:
  A. the preference of the interpreting physician
  B. the target-to-nontarget ratio
  C. the background or "noise" level
  D. all of the above

D. is correct.
Proper application of filters can reduce background noise, improve the target-to-nontarget ratio, and suppress artifacts such as the "star" effect. Trial and error will determine which groups of filters are used in any particular nuclear medicine department.

3.019 As the number of counts in a reconstructed image increases:
  A. the fewer filters will be needed
  B. the less smoothing the window function will need
  C. the more smoothing the window function will need
  D. the more filters will be needed

B. is correct.
Increased counts result in higher signal-to-noise and less smoothing in the window function is needed.

3.020 The most important factor(s) in determining quality of the tomographic image is(are):
  A. distance from collimator to the patient
  B. number of images acquired
  C. collimator resolution
  D. all of the above
  E. A and C

E. is correct.
Given an adequate number of counts, collimator to patient distance and collimator resolution are the most important factors in quality SPECT imaging. The number of images acquired is dependent on the size of the organ being imaged and resolution of the imaging system.

3.021 Pixel size is determined by:
  A. zoom factor
  B. time per image
  C. number of images acquired
  D. matrix size
  E. A and D
  F. B and D

E. is correct.
Matrix size and zoom factor work together to determine pixel size. A 64 x 64 matrix with a zoom factor of 2.0 will yield a pixel size equivalent to a 128 x 128 matrix.

3.022 Normalization of nuclear medicine images allows for:
   A. the amount of data acquisition time to be shortened
   B. simultaneous acquisitions in the posterior and anterior positions
   C. simultaneous acquisitions and processing
   D. comparison of information from different size regions of interest

D. is correct.
Normalization standardizes count information so that manipulation of data and comparison of count information from different size regions of interest (ROIs) can be accomplished. Normalization will prevent the over or underestimation of background counts based on region size.

3.023 In esophageal transit studies the computer may be used to:
   A. generate gastric emptying half-times
   B. generate time activity curves for proximal, mid, and distal regions of the esophagus
   C. evaluate the amount and distribution of gastric activity
   D. demonstrate suspected disorders of esophageal motility
   E. all of the above
   F. B and D

F. is correct.
The computer may be used to evaluate the transit time or esophageal motility in the proximal, mid, and distal end of the esophagus.

3.024 Which of the following considerations is NOT required for gastric emptying studies acquired and processed by computer?
   A. premedication with antacids
   B. correction for radioactive decay
   C. geometric correction for depth and position of stomach
   D. patient motion correction
   E. B and C

A. is correct.
The patient should be NPO ~8 hours before the exam. ROIs need to include all parts of the stomach on all images so correction for patient motion is important. The length of the exam requires decay correction and the position of the stomach requires correction for the depth and attenuation of the radiotracer in the body.

3.025 Gallbladder ejection fractions following the administration of cholecystokinin are calculated by the formula
   A. $\dfrac{\text{area under the gallbladder curve}}{\text{maximum curve height}} \times 100$
   B. $\dfrac{\text{pre CCK cts - bkgd}}{\text{post CCK cts - bkgd}} \times 100$
   C. $\dfrac{\text{pre CCK cts (-bkg) - post CCK cts (-bkg)}}{\text{pre CCK cts (-bkg)}} \times 100$
   D. $\dfrac{\text{pre CCK cts (-bkg) - post CCK cts (-bkg)}}{\text{total liver cts - bkgd}} \times 100$

C. is correct.
The gallbladder ejection fraction (GBEF) uses the pre CCK image and the post CCK images (normalized and background subtracted). Normal values are reported to be at least 35% following CCK.

3.026 Accurate assessment of cardiac ejection fractions can be obtained with a minimum of:
   A. 8 frames
   B. 16 frames
   C. 20 frames
   D. 32 frames

B. is correct.
Sixteen frames are the minimum number of frames to be acquired for an accurate assessment of cardiac ejection fraction.

3.027 In the radionuclide ventriculogram, the word image matrix which provides the best compromise between image resolution and memory required to store images is:
   A. 64 x 64
   B. 128 x 128
   C. 256 x 256
   D. none of the above

A. is correct.
There is no appreciable improvement in quantitative value by increasing matrix size. Although the image quality improves, it is really the count rate/pixel that is of value in the processing of a gated heart (or radionuclide ventriculogram) study.

3.028 The best description of a buffer is:
  A. a filter for heart rate variations
  B. a closed loop movie
  C. a temporary storage for acquired data
  D. a serial acquisition mode

C. is correct.
A buffer is a temporary storage in computer memory.

3.029 List-mode acquisitions are:
  A. a filter for heart rate variations
  B. a closed loop movie
  C. a temporary storage for acquired data
  D. a serial acquisition mode

D. is correct.
List-mode records each X, Y, Z, and R-wave trigger in a serial or list manner. It is advantageous for cardiac irregularities, but requires large amounts of memory and disk space.

3.030 The calculation of Effective Renal Plasma Flow (ERPF) and Excretory Index (EI) can be affected by all of the following considerations EXCEPT:
  A. improper dilution of the standard or samples
  B. time of data acquisition
  C. omitting the background subtraction
  D. delay in withdrawing blood sample
  E. all of the above
  F. B and C

E is correct.
All of the above can affect the calculation of ERPF or EI . Improper dilution can result in inaccurate ERPF measurements; data acquisition should be started at the time of injection to mark the arrival of the bolus in the renal region; omitting the background subtraction can overestimate the total excretion and affect the excretory index; and the blood sample should be withdrawn within 45 minutes.

3.031 In general, the number of images acquired in a 360 degree SPECT acquisition is related to the size of the organ being imaged and the resolution of the imaging system.
  A. true
  B. false

A. is correct.
The larger the organ being imaged, the more images are required to reduce the streak artifact. The better the resolution of the tomographic imaging system in use, the greater the number of images that need to be acquired.

3.032 Patient motion is one of the most common artifacts on SPECT studies. The most effective way for the technologist to detect motion is to:
  A. use a filter
  B. evaluate the raw planar images in cine format
  C. ask the patient if they moved
  D. subtract a larger area of background

B. is correct.
The images can be evaluated in cine format before the patient is taken off the imaging table.

SECTION 4: PATIENT CARE

TUTORIAL

As a member of the health care team, the nuclear medicine technologist plays an important role in helping to deliver diagnostic images that will affect a patient's care as determined by the physician. The technologist should have input into the scheduling of patient examinations in the department to insure that studies are performed in the appropriate sequence. Requisitions should be checked carefully for patient name, referring physician's name, pertinent history, and possible diagnosis. All of these will assist the technologist in assuring that the study ordered is indicated for the clinical question to be answered. Notice should be made of how the patient will travel to the department, whether oxygen will be needed, and what considerations might need to be made for each individual patient to insure the safety of that patient while in the department.

The nuclear medicine technologist should assess each patient who arrives in the department as to physical condition, whether or not the patient is in pain, and if the patient is able to lie still and flat for the examination, if required. In the absence of that patient's nurse, it is up to the technologist to observe any changes in that patient's condition. Being aware of changes in vital signs are important indicators for the patient's well-being.

In addition to the patient's physical or objective signs, subjective symptoms, such as fear, pain, apprehension, and nausea also need to be observed and dealt with. It is much easier to perform an examination on a patient who feels you have his/her best interest at heart. Gaining the confidence of the patient should be the first step of any procedure that is performed.

The preparation and administration of radiopharmaceuticals is a critical task that the nuclear medicine technologist should pay special heed to. The U.S. Nuclear Regulatory Commission defines situations of misadministration and the mechanisms for reporting a misadministration, if one occurs. The process of venipuncture should be taken seriously, and skill should be developed to prevent injury to the patient.

Patient safety is an important consideration when you are moving a patient, but it is also important to learn the proper way to move a patient for your own safety as well. In addition, proper body mechanics will make your job easier and safer for both you and your patient. The environment of health care has always been concerned with asepsis and sterile technique, but the increase in the occurrence of hepatitis B and the HIV virus have made universal precautions a necessity for the safety of everyone involved in the care and treatment of patients.

Convulsions, seizures, hemorrhage, and respiratory and cardiac arrest are among the emergency situations for which you should be prepared. The location of the emergency cart and a knowledge of what instruments and drugs are available should be a part of every technologist's initial introduction to the department. A good way to become familiar with the emergency cart is to participate in the regular checks for expired or missing drugs and equipment.

Being alert to the concerns of your patient and being aware of the special needs of each individual who comes to your department is an important responsibility of the nuclear medicine technologist. Participation in the management of each patient beyond performing their study and providing diagnostic information is important in the evaluation of the quality and appropriateness of the procedures performed. Quality assurance in patient care is everyone's responsibility and helps in decreasing errors and increasing quality patient care.

4.001   Although part of your hospital orientation will include fire safety, it is your personal responsibility to know location and information concerning which of the following?
  1. fire extinguishers
  2. fire alarms
  3. fire doors
  4. shut-off valves
A. all of these
B. 1 and 2
C. 3 and 4
D. none of these

A. is correct.
Healthcare workers must be familiar with the fire plan for the hospital, including evacuation from your area and one alternate route. In addition, have a general knowledge of your facility's floor plan, being certain of location of fire alarms, fire extinguishers, and fire doors.

4.002   When transporting a patient by stretcher, the use of safety belts or side rails is required:
A. when restraint has been ordered by the physician
B. for patients who are uncooperative or unconscious
C. for children
D. for all patients
E. both B and C

D. is correct.
Stretchers are equipped with safety straps or side rails to ensure that patients will not fall or attempt to slide off stretcher without assistance. This safety practice is followed without exception.

4.003   Patients who suffer from orthopnea need to have:
A. padding under bony prominences
B. their heads elevated in order to breathe
C. the feet elevated to avoid pain
D. restraints applied to avoid falls
E. a skin graft

B. is correct.
Orthopnea is the ability to breathe easily only in the upright position, so elevation of the patient's head allows for easier breathing.

4.004   A patient suffering from severe abdominal pain will be most comfortable when:
A. the head is elevated
B. a bolster is placed under the knees
C. the head is lower than the feet
D. placed in the prone position
E. both A and B

E. is correct.
Addition of a bolster under the knees of a supine patient relieves lumbosacral stress and strain to the abdomen.

4.005   In case of electrical fire, which of the following fire extinguishers can be used to extinguish the fire?
  1. CO_2 foam
  2. Halon
  3. H_2O
  4. Chemical
A. 1, 2, and 3
B. 1 and 2
C. 3 and 4
D. all of the above

B. is correct.
In case of electrical fire, use CO_2 or Halon fire extinguishers. H_2O and chemical extinguishers increase the hazard of electrical shock.

4.006   When placing patients in the supine position, consideration should be taken for which of the following conditions?
A. patients with dyspnea or orthopnea
B. patients who are nauseated
C. patients with abdominal pain
D. A and B
E. all of the above

E. is correct.
Patients with dyspnea or orthopnea are unable to lie supine. Patients who are nauseated need to have heads of beds elevated to prevent aspiration of vomitus if patient vomits. Patients with abdominal pain need to have their head elevated and bolster paced under knees to relieve strain on the abdomen.

4.007 Which of the following are not microorganisms?
A. bacteria
B. fungi
C. vectors
D. protozoans
E. viruses

C. is correct.
A vector is an animal in whose body an infectious organism develops or multiplies before becoming infective in a new host.

4.008 A fomite is:
A. a microorganism
B. a contaminated object
C. an insect that transmits disease
D. an antiseptic
E. a means of airborne contamination

B. is correct.
An object that has been in contact with pathogenic organisms is called a fomite.

4.009 Which of the following statements is NOT appropriate with regard to handling patient items?
A. no item should ever be used for more than one patient without being laundered first
B. bags containing badly soiled or contaminated linen should be marked before sending them to the laundry
C. used linens should be rolled into a loose ball before placing them in the hamper
D. soiled linens should be thoroughly shaken before placing them in the hamper
E. used linens are considered contaminated even when no stain is apparent

D. is correct.
To prevent airborne contamination, fold the edges of linens to the middle without shaking or flapping sheets.

4.010 Under the system of body system precautions, the health care worker who is trained to start or discontinue IV's:
A. must wear gloves
B. must wear gloves only when starting IV's
C. must wear gloves only when removing IV's
D. must wear sterile gloves

A. is correct.
Gloves should be worn when it is likely that hands will be in contact with body substances (blood, urine, feces, wound drainage, oral secretions, sputum, vomitus).

4.011 Which of the following is the best way the healthcare worker can prevent the spread of microorganism from one patient to another?
A. by using adequate hand washing
B. by working through an infection-review committee
C. by using isolation techniques
D. by teaching patients good hygiene practices

A. is correct.
The single most effective means of preventing the spread of infection is hand washing.

4.012 All of the following are essential components of the hand washing procedure EXCEPT:
A. friction
B. running water
C. foot operated water controls
D. cleansing agent

C. is correct.
Water controls may be foot-operated, knee-operated, or hand-operated.

4.013 Scrubbing with soap and water is an example of:
A chemical removal of bacteria
B mechanical removal of bacteria
C personal hygiene
D all of the above

D. is correct.

4.014 Conditions ideal for the growth of pathogenic bacteria are:
   A. light and moisture
   B. rough, dry surfaces
   C. darkness and dry surfaces
   D. warmth and moisture

D. is correct.
Pathogens can thrive any place which provides moisture, nutrients, and a suitable temperature, all of which are found in the human body.

4.015 Hand washing when caring for the patient in isolation is creating:
   A. a barrier
   B. a reservoir
   C. a sterile field
   D. surgical asepsis

A. is correct.
A barrier is any technique performed to intervene in transmission of disease.

4.016 General principles of environmental asepsis apply to all of the following EXCEPT:
   A. always clean from the least contaminated area toward the more contaminated area
   B. always clean from the top down
   C. avoid raising dust
   D. always clean from the more contaminated area toward the least contaminated area

D. is correct.
Cleaning from an area of lesser contamination helps to contain the contamination rather than spread it.

4.017 AIDS, which is caused by Human Immunodeficiency Virus, may be transmitted by all of the following means EXCEPT:
   A. blood to blood contact
   B. sexual contact
   C. casual contact
   D. perinatal exposure

C. is correct.
Aids can only be transmitted by sexual contact, by contaminated needles, or by infected mother to fetus.

4.018 Serious viral diseases, which may be spread through infected blood and body fluids, include:
   A. tuberculosis
   B. Hepatitis B
   C. AIDS
   D. dysentery
   E. B and C
   F. all of the above

E. is correct.
Both TB and dysentery are transmitted by bacteria.

4.019 Procedures that generate splashing blood and body fluids require which of the following protective attire?
   A. gloves
   B. masks
   C. protective eyewear
   D. gowns
   E. all of the above

E. is correct.
Gloves protect hands from contact with body substances, gowns protect clothing when it is likely to be soiled, and masks and protective eyewear protect eyes and mucus membranes which can be contaminated with splashes of blood and body fluids.

4.020 When a physician orders "NPO" for a patient, this means that:
   A. all urine samples must be saved
   B. only water and ice chips are to given by mouth
   C. intravenous therapy is to be given
   D. nothing is to be given by mouth
   E. the patient may walk to the bathroom

D. is correct.
NPO is the abbreviation for nothing by mouth. (literally "non per os")

4.021 When checking a patient for signs of cyanosis, one should note the coloration of the:
  A. eyes
  B. lips and nail beds
  C. palms of the hands and soles of the feet
  D. cheeks
  E. forehead and neck

B. is correct.
Cyanosis is bluish discoloration of the skin and nail beds, due to lack of oxygen in the blood.

4.022 The term "diaphoretic" means:
  A. cool
  B. feverish
  C. cyanotic
  D. sweaty

D. is correct.
Diaphoresis is the secretion of sweat, especially the profuse secretion associated with an elevated body temperature, physical exertion, exposure to heat, and mental or emotional stress.

4.023 Blood pressure can most accurately be defined as:
  A. oxygen concentration in the blood
  B. pressure of blood on the walls of veins
  C. pressure in the left ventricle during contraction
  D. pressure of blood on the walls of arteries

D. is correct.
The pressure in the aorta and large arteries of a healthy young adult is approximately 120 mm Hg during systole and 70 mm Hg in diastole.

4.024 The diaphragm of the stethoscope should be placed over which artery to measure blood pressure in the arm?
  A. radial
  B. brachial
  C. femoral
  D. carotid

B. is correct.
Palpating the antecubital space for the brachial pulse and placing the diaphragm of the stethoscope over this area while placing the earpieces in the ears to listen to the blood pressure is proper technique.

4.025 Treating an item as to make it completely free of all organisms and their spores is called:
  A. asepsis
  B. disinfection
  C. microbial dilution
  D. sterilization
  E. decontamination

B. is correct.
Disinfection is the process of killing pathogenic organisms or of rendering them inert.

4.026 Which of the following is the most common sterilization process used in hospitals?
  A. boiling water
  B. steam under pressure
  C. ethylene oxide gas
  D. sporicidal chemicals

B. is correct.
Autoclaving is steam under pressure. This method is most frequently used to sterilize items in hospitals.

4.027 A plastic tubing to an instrument must be sterilized. The best method to use would be:
  A. boiling water
  B. steam under pressure
  C. ethylene oxide gas
  D. sporicidal chemicals

C. is correct.
Items that can be damaged by high degrees of heat or have cement used in their construction must be sterilized by ethylene oxide gas.

4.028 Gas sterilization is used primarily for all of the following EXCEPT:
  A. cystoscopic and fiberoptic instruments
  B. thermometers, blood pressure cuffs and stethoscopes
  C. metal instruments
  D. plastic and rubber items

C. is correct.
Metal instruments may be sterilized using steam heat.

4.029 In preparing to draw solution into a syringe, you are not certain whether or not you have brushed the needle against the outside of the needle cover. What guideline should you use as a basis for action?
  A. microorganisms travel rapidly along any moisture through a wicking action
  B. any item to be sterilized must be completely clean
  C. anything outside is considered to be unsterile
  D. if in doubt about the sterility of an item, consider it unsterile

D. is correct.
When in doubt, throw it out.

4.030 A metal instrument set must be sterilized. Which of the following techniques would be most appropriate?
  A. boiling water
  B. steam under pressure
  C. ethylene oxide gas
  D. sporicidal chemicals

B. is correct.
Metal instruments would not be harmed by steam.

4.031 Drugs given prior to surgery in certain procedures for the purpose of suppressing secretions belong to the category known as:
  A. analgesics
  B. anticholinergics
  C. anticoagulants
  D. antihistamines
  E. anti emetics

B. is correct.
Anticholinergic drugs decrease gastric, bronchial salivary secretions, and decrease perspiration.

4.032 A drug usually takes effect most rapidly when administered:
  A. orally
  B. subcutaneously
  C. intramuscularly
  D. intradermally
  E. intravenously

E. is correct.
Drugs administered IV are immediately transported to organs and tissues which offers rapid response to the medication.

4.033 When extravasation occurs as a result of an intravenous injection, the treatment involves:
  A. medication
  B. dry heat
  C. moist heat
  D. cold packs
  E. massage

C. is correct.
Hot packs or moist heat can help alleviate pain and expedite absorption of fluids accidentally injected into the tissues.

4.034 Failure to apply pressure to the vein after discontinuing an IV may result in:
  A. extravasation
  B. infiltration
  C. coagulation
  D. hematoma
  E. laceration

D. is correct.
Blood may leak into the tissues around the site of the IV upon the removal of the needle from the vein. Pressure on the site will cause the blood to clot.

4.035 The most common site for intravenous injection is:
  A. the antecubital vein
  B. the brachial artery
  C. the radial artery
  D. the saphenous vein
  E. the pulmonary vein

A. is correct.
The antecubital veins on each arm are large enough and near enough to the surface to be easily seen, palpated, and punctured.

4.036 Drugs that relax the walls of blood vessels, permitting a greater flow of blood are:
  A. cardiac stimulants
  B. hyperglycemics
  C. antiemetics
  D. vasodilators

D. is correct.
Vasodilators relax the vessel walls allowing a greater flow of blood through the vessels.

4.037 All parenteral medications are given using strict:
  A. medical aseptic technique
  B. surgical aseptic technique
  C. isolation technique
  D. reverse isolation technique

B. is correct.
Strict surgical asepsis is necessary to prevent introducing organisms into underlying tissues during parenteral administration of drugs.

4.038 When preparing a parenteral injection, it is essential to keep which of the following areas sterile?
  A. top of the plunger
  B. needle shaft and tip
  C. exterior of ampule or vial
  D. outside barrel portion of syringe

B. is correct.
The needle shaft and tip, along with the inside of the barrel of the syringe and the plunger must remain sterile to prevent transmission of organisms into body tissues.

4.039 Which of the following types of medication may cause respiratory depression?
  A. anticholinergics
  B. diuretics
  C. tranquilizer/sedatives
  D. antihistamines
  E. antagonists

C. is correct.
These drugs cause CNS depression which includes respiratory depression, since the respirations are controlled by centers in the brain.

4.040 Drugs that prevent or counteract respiratory depression and other depressive effects of morphine and related drugs are:
  A. radioactive isotopes
  B. antiperistaltics
  C. narcotic antagonists
  D. cathartics

C. is correct.
Antagonists reverse the effect of the drugs.

4.041 The technique in which a vein is punctured to withdraw a specimen of blood, to instill a medication, or start an intravenous infusion is:
  A. arterial puncture
  B. skin puncture
  C. venipuncture
  D. phlebotomy

C. is correct.
Venipuncture is the technique used to enter the vein. Phlebotomy is the incision of a vein for letting of blood, as in collecting blood from a donor.

4.042   Which vein of the forearm is most frequently used for venipuncture?
  A. femoral
  B. superior vena cava
  C. median cubital
  D. carotid

C. is correct.
The median cubital vein is often visible and palpable in the adult patient.

4.043   While performing a venipuncture, transfixation can result in:
  A. formation of a deep hematoma
  B. syncope
  C. hemoconcentration
  D. nausea and vomiting

A. is correct.
Transfixation occurs when the needle goes through both sides of the vein allowing blood to escape from the underside of the vein into surrounding tissues.

4.044   If the patient continues to bleed once the needle is removed:
  A. order a type and cross match
  B. reapply the tourniquet
  C. apply pressure to the site with a gauze pad until bleeding stops
  D. gently massage the arm from wrist to elbow

C. is correct.
Applying pressure will prevent blood from escaping the vein.

4.045   When one palpates thrombosed veins, they:
  A. lack resilience
  B. feel cord like
  C. roll easily
  D. all of the above

D. is correct.
Hard, sclerosed veins lack a bouncy, spongy feel and will roll easily under the skin.

4.046   Which of the following incidents should be reported as a body fluid exposure?
  A. blood splashed on intact skin of the arm
  B. a scratch to the hand from a clean needle
  C. spray of blood or urine in the eye
  D. spray of blood onto an impervious lab coat

C. is correct.
The eye splashed with body fluids can cause direct access into blood vessels through mucus membranes.

4.047   Materials that should be considered potentially infectious for the organisms that transmit hepatitis B or AIDS include all of the following EXCEPT:
  A. gauze caked with dried blood from an arterial puncture procedure
  B. urine dipsticks
  C. used phlebotomy needles
  D. fluids from a suction canister in the intensive care unit
  E. blood-soaked paper towels used in cleaning up a spill

B. is correct.
These items (unused urine dipsticks) have not touched body substances or fluids.

4.048   Protective personal equipment should be chosen to protect skin and clothing from possible contamination. Protective personal equipment includes:
  A. gloves when handling body fluids
  B. gowns or lab coats when splashing of fluids of clothes is expected
  C. mask and goggles if spraying of body fluids on the face is expected
  D. CPR masks if an emergency CPR is performed
  E. all of the above

E. is correct.

4.049 The bevel of the needle should be in which position before entering a vein?
   A. facing down
   B. facing toward the side
   C. facing upward
   D. it really does not matter, as long as the venipuncture is performed quickly

C. is correct.
With the bevel up, there is less chance of transfixation of a vein.

4.050 Which of the following is not classified as a barrier precaution?
   A. HBV vaccine
   B. gloves
   C. goggles
   D. gown or apron

A. is correct.
HBV is the hepatitis B virus vaccine. A series of three doses is recommended to achieve immunity.

4.051 This recent OSHA regulation requires all health care personnel at risk for exposure to _____ to receive vaccination.
   A. hepatitis A virus
   B. hepatitis B virus
   C. hepatitis C virus
   D. hepatitis Delta virus

B. is correct.

4.052 If a technologist is unsure about performing a study that is ordered on a patient's requisition, the technologist should:
   A. confirm the study with the patient
   B. confirm the study with the floor nurse
   C. obtain clarification from the requesting party
   D. obtain clarification from the nuclear medicine physician
   E. C or D
   F. none of the above

E. is correct.
If clarification on a study is needed, obtain it from either the requesting physician or the nuclear medicine physician.

4.053 What should be done if a nursing patient is to be studied in the nuclear medicine department?
   A. the study should be postponed indefinitely
   B. the woman should be advised to cease nursing for 24 hours prior to testing
   C. the woman should be advised to cease nursing for 24 hours after testing
   D. an informed consent is needed for nursing patients

C. is correct.
For studies done using ^{99m}Tc, a nursing patient may collect breast milk for the 24 hours following the exam and let it decay to background.

4.054 What is the danger in imaging patients in the standing position?
   A. one cannot get the camera close to the patient's surface
   B. the patient may become hypotensive and fall
   C. the camera does not operate properly and images will demonstrate asymmetry
   D. the patient may contaminate the collimator

B. is correct.
A patient should never be imaged in the standing position; the patient may become hypotensive and fall. Upright images may be taken in the sitting position.

SECTION 5: RADIOPHARMACY

TUTORIAL

Preparation and familiarity with the radiopharmaceuticals that are used in the nuclear medicine laboratory are an important part of the technologist's responsibility. A radiopharmaceutical is a radioactive drug that is intended for human administration for diagnostic or therapeutic purposes and as such comes under the jurisdiction of both the Nuclear Regulatory Commission (NRC) and the Food and Drug Administration (FDA).

The quality of the radiopharmaceutical or radiopharmaceutical kit is the responsibility of the manufacturer, but the final preparation, and therefore the quality assurance procedures for that final product, lies with the nuclear medicine technologist or radiopharmacist preparing and dispensing those preparations.

Equipment and instrumentation used for assay should be calibrated and tested regularly and all personnel should have a basic understanding of the radiopharmakinetics, physiology, and preparation techniques involved in the preparation of radiopharmaceuticals.

Aseptic technique will assure that the sterility and apyrogenicity of the preparations is maintained. Radiopharmaceuticals (e.g., ^{99m}Tc pertechnatate) may be instilled in the bladder or into the eye as well as being injected into the body. All procedures require the agent to be sterile. Eluents from the ^{99}Mo/^{99m}Tc generator must be checked each time they are eluted for radionuclidic purity ("Moly breakthrough") and aluminum breakthrough. Radiochemical purity is checked using chromatography.

Dose preparation should include the repetition of certain steps regardless of the number of doses drawn. Each time a dose is draw the following should be observed:

1. Examine the label, type of radiopharmaceutical (Is it appropriate for the study being performed?), and date of expiration (or time of preparation).

2. Examine the vial briefly for unusual changes in color or precipitates. (If changes are observed, THROW IT OUT!)

3. Note the concentration and time of assay.

4. Determine the volume to be withdrawn into the syringe.

5. Enter information on data sheets.

6. Draw the dose into a pre-labeled syringe (radiopharmaceutical, amount in mCi, and date).

Familiarity with biorouting and excretion routes will assist the technologist in trouble-shooting artifacts that may appear to be due to radiopharmaceutical preparation or are a part of the normal accumulation of the radiopharmaceutical.

5.001 The body weight of a standardized man for dose calculations is based on the _____kg man model.
  A. 50
  B. 70
  C. 100
  D. 150
  E. 175

B. is correct.
70 kg is equal to 154 pounds and is used as the standard for dose calculations.

5.002 The concentration (C) of a radiopharmaceutical is given by which of the following?
  A. C = activity (A) x volume (V)
  B. C = A/V
  C. C = V/A
  D. none of the above

B. is correct.
Concentration is expressed as the activity (in mCi) per unit volume (in ml).

5.003 A vial contains 250 uCi of 111In in 5 ml of fluid. The concentration is:
  A. 250 uCi/ml
  B. 25 uCi/ml
  C. 50 mCi/ml
  D. 50 uCi/ml

D. is correct.
250uCi/5 ml = 50 uCi/ml; the concentration of 111In in the vial.

5.004 A vial contains ^{99m}Tc at a concentration of 58 mCi / ml. A dose of 15 mCi is desired. How many ml should be withdrawn into the syringe? (i.e., What volume is required?)
  A. 0.26 ml
  B. 2.6 ml
  C. 0.39 ml
  D. 3.9 ml
  E. 0.87 ml

A. is correct.
$V = A / C$ or $V = \dfrac{15\ mCi}{58\ mCi/ml} = 0.26\ ml$
or put "what you want" over "what you've got" to get the volume.

5.005 A vial contains 350 mCi of ^{99m}Tc in 30 ml of fluid. What is the concentration?
  A. 11.7 mCi/ml
  B. 1.17 mCi/ml
  C. 0.86 mCi/ml
  D. 0.09 mCi/ml

A. is correct.
C = A/V = 350 mCi/30 ml = 11.7 mCi/ml

5.006 180 mCi in 10 ml is added to 100 ml. The resulting concentration is:
  A. 0.16 mCi/ml
  B. 0.18 mCi/ml
  C. 1.6 mCi/ml
  D. 1.8 mCi/ml
  E. 18 mCi/ml

C. is correct.
The new volume is 110 ml, so C = 180 mCi / 110 ml = 1.6 mCi/ml.

5.007 A vial contains 260 mCi in 20 ml of fluid. How many ml should be withdrawn to obtain 20 mCi?
  A. 0.07
  B. 0.65
  C. 1.30
  D. 1.54
  E. none of the above

D. is correct.
The concentration in the vial is 260mCi/20 ml or 13 mCi/ml. To obtain a 20 mCi dose, 1.54 ml need to be withdrawn. (20/13 = 1.54)

5.008 The half-life of a radioactive substance is the time it takes:
   A. to decay to one-half its original activity
   B. to deliver one-half of its radiation dose
   C. for the number of radioactive nuclei to decrease by one-half
   D. A and B
   E. A, B, and C

E. is correct.

5.009 The decay constant is
   A. the fraction of nuclei which decay per unit time
   B. the rate of radioactive decay
   C. the rate at which radiation dose is delivered
   D. A and B
   E. A and C

A. is correct.

5.010 P-32 has a half-life of 14.3 days. A sample has an original activity of 200 mCi. How much will be left after 3 days? (decay factor = .8644)
   A. 173 mCi
   B. 175 mCi
   C. 179 mCi
   D. 184 mCi

A. is correct.
200 mCi x .8644 = 173 mCi

5.011 A 57Co capsule is dissolved in 50 ml of water. How many ml should be withdrawn to make a 10% standard?
   A. 2.5
   B. 5.0
   C. 10.0
   D. 25.0

B. is correct.
50 ml x .10 = 5 ml

5.012 A pediatric dose must be prepared for a patient undergoing a bone scan. It has been determined that the patient should receive 67% of the standard adult dose of 20 mCi. What is the dose in mCi that the patient should receive?
   A. 6.7 mCi
   B. 9.25 mCi
   C. 13.4 mCi
   D. 18.0 mCi

C. is correct.
20 mCi x .67 = 13.4 mCi

5.013 I-123 has a half-life of 13 hours. A sample of the material has an activity of 5.6 mCi at noon today. What was its activity at noon yesterday? (decay factor = 3.526)
   A. 10 mCi
   B. 15 mCi
   C. 20 mCi
   D. 25 mCi

C. is correct.
5.6mCi X 3.526 = 20mCi at noon yesterday.

5.014 A radiopharmaceutical kit is prepared at 11:00 AM with 3 ml of ^{99m}Tc pertechnatate from generate eluate that is calibrated for 600 mCi/5 ml at 6:00 AM. How much activity will the kit contain? (The 5 hour decay factor is 0.561)
- A. 1011 mCi
- B. 360 mCi
- C. 202 mCi
- D. 120 mCi
- E. 67 mCi

C. is correct.
At 11:00 AM the concentration will be 67 mCi/ml. Using 3 ml will put 202 mCi of activity in the kit.

5.015 On April 4, a radiopharmaceutical is received and calibrated at 150 uCi/ml. What is the concentration in uCi/ml, on April 20? (T1/2 = 8 days)
- A. 150
- B. 75
- C. 50
- D. 37.5
- E. 18.75

C. is correct.
After 1 half-life (April 12), there is 75 uCi/ml; after a second half-life decay (April 20), there will be 37.5 uCi/ml left.

5.016 A 10 mCi source of 201 Tl thallous chloride in a volume of 5 ml, calibrated for June 10, at 12 noon EST, was received on June 9. What would be the activity on June 9, at 1:00 PM EST? (pre-calibration decay factor for 25 hours = 1.26)
- A. 1.6 mCi/ml
- B. 2.52 mCi/ml
- C. 7.9 mCi/ml
- D. 12.6 mCi/ml

B. is correct.
Final activity = initial activity x decay factor
FA = 10 mCi x 1.26 = 12.6 mCi/5 ml or 2.52 mCi/ml

5.017 210uCi of 131 I hippuran is to be used on May 3. There was 300 uCi on the date of the assay, April 29. Is the activity present on May 3 acceptable for the prescribed dose? (decay factor = 0.651)
- A. no, because the activity remaining is less than 50% of the prescribed dose
- B. yes, because the activity remaining is greater than the prescribed dose
- C. yes, because the activity remaining is within 10 % of the prescribed dose
- D. as long as a diagnostic study can be obtained, the dose is irrelevant
- E. none of the above

C. is correct.
FA(final activity) = 300 uCi x 0.651 (five day decay factor for 131 I) = 195.3 uCi on May 3 (within +/- 10% of 210 uCi)

5.018 If the radioactivity of a ^{99m}Tc sample is 40 mCi at 8:00 AM, what will the activity of the sample be at 8:00 PM?
- A. 80 mCi
- B. 20 mCi
- C. 15 mCi
- D. 10 mCi

D. is correct.
The half-life of ^{99m}Tc is 6 hours. After 2 half lives, or 12 hours, the activity will be 10 mCi. (After one half-life, the activity is 20 mCi).

5.019 In a ^{99m}Tc/^{99}Mo radionuclide generator, the material onto which the parent radionuclide is adsorbed is:
- A. alumina
- B. aluminum
- C. aluminum hydroxide
- D. aluminum ion

A. is correct.
The ^{99}Mo activity is bound to an alumina (Al^2O^3) column.

5.020 After equilibrium has been disturbed by elution, a radionuclide generation will return to equilibrium in about:
   A. 4 daughter half-lives
   B. 4 parent half-lives
   C. 2 daughter half-lives
   D. 2 parent half-lives

A. is correct.
For the ^{99}Mo/^{99m}Tc generator system this will be accomplished in about 24 hours. (T1/2 ^{99m}Tc = 6 hours)

5.021 Aluminum breakthrough in ^{99}Mo/^{99m}Tc generators can be a problem because the aluminum ions can:
   A. cause the eluent to be nonsterile
   B. cause a low grade fever in patients who receive radiopharmaceuticals prepared with the ^{99m}Tc eluate
   C. affect the biodistribution and tagging reactions
   D. deliver an unnecessarily high dose to patients receiving preparations with the ^{99m}Tc eluate

C. is correct.
Alumina breakthrough from the generator column is a chemical impurity and can affect the biodistribution of radiopharmaceuticals prepared from the ^{99m}Tc eluate.

5.022 The USP (United States Pharmacopoeia) has established a maximum limit of _____ Al^{+3}/ml eluate.
   A. 0.15 ug
   B. 1.0 ug
   C. 1.5 ug
   D. 10 ug
   E. 15 ug

D. is correct.
No more than 10 ug of Al^{+3} per ml of eluate is acceptable.

5.023 The presence of aluminum ions in the ^{99m}Tc eluate is an example of a:
   A. radionuclidic impurity
   B. radiochemical impuriity
   C. colloidal impurity
   D. pyrogenic impurity
   E. chemical impurity

E. is correct.
Non-radioactive impurities in radiopharmaceutical preparations that can interfere with the labeling of pharmaceuticals or adversely affect the patient, are chemical impurities.

5.024 A patient injected with ^{99m}Tc MDP and scanned 2 hours post injection demonstrated activity in the liver. This was most likely due to:
   A. scanning too soon after injection of MDP
   B. extravasation of the dose
   C. presence of ^{99m}Tc-tin colloids
   D. presence of free or unbound ^{99m}Tc pertechnatate

C. is correct.
Excess stannous ion which is used in kit preparation as a reducing agent, may contribute to the formation of ^{99m}Tc-tin colloids which will result in liver uptake.

5.025 A bone agent was prepared at 7:30 AM and a patient dose administered at 1:00 PM. The patient was scanned 2 hours post injection and the bone scan shows activity in the salivary glands and stomach. This activity is most likely due to:
   A. scanning too soon after injection of MDP
   B. extravasation of the dose
   C. presence of ^{99m}Tc-tin colloids
   D. presence of free or unbound ^{99m}Tc pertechnatate

D. is correct.
The presence of free ^{99m}Tc pertechnatate will bioroute to the thyroid, salivary glands, stomach (gastric mucosa), and choroid plexes.

5.026 Following the administration of a radiopharmaceutical for a diagnostic imaging study, the patient develops a high fever and chills. This is most likely a _____ reaction.
   A. radiation
   B. bronchogenic
   C. pyrogenic
   D. cardiovascular
   E. anaphylactic

C. is correct.
A pyrogenic reaction is one in which a fever is produced. The limulus amebocyte lysate test is used by manufacturers to test for the presence of gram-negative bacterial endotoxins. Aseptic technique must be used when reconstituting the drugs to insure that sterility and apyrogenicity are maintained prior to patient administration.

5.027 The remaining ^{99m}Tc that remains untagged after the preparation of ^{99m}Tc MDP are:
   A. radionuclidic impurities
   B. radiochemical imuriities
   C. colloidal impurities
   D. pyrogenic impurities
   E. chemical impurities

B. is correct.
The presence of free ^{99m}Tc (untagged) in a kit preparation represents a radiochemical impurity.

5.028 The presence of ^{99}Mo in the ^{99m}Tc pertechnatate eluate is a:
   A. radionuclidic impurity
   B. radiochemical impuriity
   C. colloidal impurity
   D. pyrogenic impurity
   E. chemical impurity

A. is correct.
Radionuclidic purity is the amount of the total radioactivity present in a sample that is in the stated radionuclide. The presence of an impurity such as ^{99}Mo can significantly increase the radiation dose to the patient as well as affect image quality.

5.029 In performing a molybdenum 99 ("Moly") break through test, a technologist assays 102 uCi of ^{99}Mo in 950 mCi of ^{99m}Tc pertechnatate. This assay is _____ the allowable limits of _____ uCi ^{99}Mo/mCi ^{99m}Tc for radionuclidic impurities set by the NRC.
   A. outside of; 0.10
   B. outside of; 0.15
   C. within; 0.10
   D. within; 0.15
   E. the same as; 0.10

D. is correct.
The Nuclear Regulatory Commission allowable radionuclidic impurities in ^{99m}Tc pertechnatate for ^{99}Mo is less than 0.15 uCi of Mo per mCi of ^{99m}Tc. ^{99}Mo is the parent in the ^{99}Mo / ^{99m}Tc generator system and is a likely contaminant of the eluate. It is easily assayed for using a dose calibrator because of the differences in energies; 740 keV for ^{99}Mo and 140 keV for ^{99m}Tc.

5.030 A ^{99}Mo / ^{99m}Tc generator is eluted at 2:00 PM for an emergency study and is assayed. The technologist records 47 uCi of ^{99}Mo in 270 mCi of ^{99m}Tc pertechnatate. What should happen next?
   A. the eluate should be tested for the presence of aluminum ion
   B. no testing is necessary for emergency studies performed during the work day; the dose should be drawn for the study
   C. the ^{99}Mo break through is greater than allowable by the NRC and should not be used for patient administration
   D. the radiation safety officer should be notified
   E. B and D

C. is correct.
47uCi/270mCi = .174uCi ^{99}Mo/ mCi ^{99m}Tc is greater than the allowable limit (^{99}Mo < 0.15 uCi/mCi ^{99M}Tc). Each elution of the generator must be tested and be less than the allowable limit for radionuclidic impurities set by the NRC (Nuclear Regulatory Commission).

5.031 Records established on April 1, 1996, on ^{99}Mo breakthrough tests on elutions from the ^{99}Mo / ^{99m}Tc generator elutions must be kept for a period of _____ year(s), or until April, _____.
   A. one; 1997
   B. two; 1998
   C. three; 1999
   D. four; 2000
   E. five; 2001

C. is correct.
NRC requires that records from each elution of the generator be kept for a period of three years.

5.032 Which elution process is most commonly used in a ^{99}Mo/^{99m}Tc generator?
   A. distillation
   B. ion exchange
   C. solvent extraction
   D. precipitation

B. is correct.
Elution of the generator with normal saline results in the ^{99m}Tc sodium pertechnatate dissolved in the normal saline and the parent ^{99}Mo remaining on the column. The differences in chemistry allow the daughter to be separated from the parent.

5.033 Persantine (dipyridamole), used during myocardial imaging, acts as a(n):
   A. anti-inflammatory agent
   B. vasoconstrictor
   C. anticoagulant
   D. vasodilator

D. is correct.
I.V. Dipyridamole is a potent coronary artery vasodilator.

5.034 Persantine inhibits the uptake of:
   A. theophylline
   B. beta blockers
   C. adenosine
   D. dipyridamole

C. is correct.
Oral dipyridamole inhibits the metabolism of adenosine.

5.035 The vasodilatory effects of Persantine (dipyridamole) are reversed by administering:
   A. aminophylline
   B. adenosine
   C. theophylline
   D. dipyridamole

A. is correct.
Intravenous aminophylline has been shown to reverse the pharmacologic actions of I.V. dipyridamole within approximately one minute after injection.

5.036 Which of the following may cause malabsorption of vitamin B_{12}?
   1. antibiotics
   2. steroids
   3. excessive alcohol consumption
   A. 1 and 2
   B. 1 and 3
   C. 2 and 3
   D. 1, 2, and 3

B. is correct.
Long term use of antibiotics and excessive alcohol consumption can cause intestinal malabsorption by impairing some of the mucosal absorptive sites in the ileum.

5.037 Which of the following medications enhance 99mTc concentration in the gastric mucosa?
   A. cimetidine
   B. lasix
   C. pyrophosphate
   D. Persantine

A. is correct.
The administration of cimetidine may decrease the release of pertechnatate from the ectopic mucosa into the bowel.

5.038 Which of the following statements is NOT true regarding the labeling of 111In oxine white blood cells (WBC)?
  A. All traces of plasma should be removed before labeling.
  B. The In^{+3} will pass through the WBC membrane.
  C. The 111In-labeling technique requires aseptic technique.
  D. It is necessary to withdraw 30 to 50 ml of blood from the patient.

B. is correct.
The In^{+3} ion will not pass through the WBC membrane because of its electronic charge. It easily penetrates the WBC membrane when it is in the complex formed with oxines, a lipophilic agent.

5.039 The minimum number of radiolabeled particles (MAA, macroaggregated albumin) for a satisfactory lung perfusion scan is:
  A. 10,000
  B. 30,000
  C. 60,000
  D. 100,000

C. is correct.
Perfusion imaging may be satisfactorily performed with a minimum of 60,000 particles in the normal patient. Generally, between 60,000 and 150,000 particles are injected. (as many as 200,000-700,000 particles may be injected per dose). If too few particles are injected, there is a blotchy appearance to the scan.

5.040 A technologist could perform the quality control testing on MAA to include:
  A. instant thin-layer chromatography
  B. particle sizing
  C. limulus amebocyte lysate
  D. all of the above
  E. A and B only

E. is correct.
The presence of free pertechnatate can be determined using ITLC and particle sizing is conducted using a hemocytometer grid under a microscope. The limulus amebocyte lysate test is performed by the manufacturer on their products to test for pyrogenicity.

5.041 Full generation of the ^{99}Mo/^{99m}Tc column takes at least:
  A. 6 hours
  B. 12 hours
  C. 24 hours
  D. 48 hours

C. is correct.
Maximum activity is available about 24 hours after an elution and can be determined using methods of calculus and the half-lives of the parent (^{99}Mo = 66 hours) and the daughter (^{99m}Tc = 6 hours).

5.042 Adding saline to a ^{99}Mo/^{99m}Tc generator is required for which of the following?
  A. wet column
  B. dry column
  C. alumina column
  D. hot column

B. is correct.
The wet column generator contains a normal saline reservoir, while the dry column generator uses a saline charge or vial applied to an external port.

5.043 ^{99m}Tc sulfur colloid localizes in functional liver tissue as a result of:
  A. active transport
  B. phagocytosis
  C. capillary blockade
  D. cell sequestration

B. is correct.
^{99m}Tc sulfur colloid is cleared from the blood by the cells of the reticuloendothelial system which phagocytize the colloid particles.

5.044 Phosphorus 32 is best described as:
  A. an alpha emitter
  B. a gamma emitter
  C. a beta emitter
  D. a beta-gamma emitter

C. is correct.
Phosphorus 32 (P32) is a pure beta emitter which decays to S32 with the emission of a beta particle and an antineutrino and no gamma emissions.

5.045 Which of the following radionuclides is NOT routinely used for lung ventilation studies?
   A. 133Xe
   B. ^{99m}Tc DTPA aerosol
   C. 67Ga
   D. 81mKr

C. is correct.
Nebulized aerosols such as ^{99m}Tc DTPA and the inert gases, 133Xe, 127Xe (no longer available), and 81mKr, are used to study ventilation of lungs. 67Ga might be used to evaluate an inflammatory process or in staging and detecting tumors in lung tissue. In addition, 67Ga has great avidity for the Pneumocystis pneumonia.

5.046 The following occurs as filtered air is introduced into the ^{99m}Tc MAG3 reaction vial during the boiling phase:
   A. pH is stabilized
   B. reduction of the Mertiatide compound
   C. progressive formation of labeled impurities
   D. oxidation of excess stannous ions

D. is correct.
Oxygen present in the vial oxidizes remaining stannous ion to prevent the formation of lower valence states of technetium. (Lower valence states are responsible for the formation of radiochemical impurities in the preparation).

5.047 Which of the following gases is released upon adding ^{99m}Tc pertechnatate to a MAG3 reagent vial?
   A. carbon dioxide
   B. nitrogen
   C. oxygen
   D. argon

D. is correct.
Argon gas in the vial is released when the pertechnatate is added and air is withdrawn from the vial to be replaced with atmospheric air.

5.048 The stannous ion found within a reagent vial may hydrolyze to stannous hydroxide when:
   A. air is introduced
   B. water is present
   C. nitrogen escapes
   D. carbon dioxide is introduced

B. is correct.
In the presence of water (H_2O), excess stannous ion may hydrolyze to stannous hydroxide and degrade the contents of the ^{99m}Tc-labeled radiopharmaceutical kit.

5.049 Oxidation of the stannous ion occurs when:
   A. water is introduced
   B. nitrogen is introduced
   C. carbon dioxide is introduced
   D. air is introduced

D. is correct.
The introduction of air (oxygen) into the reaction vial may oxidize the stannous ion to stannic ion (Sn^{+4}), which is ineffective as a reducing agent.

5.050 A common contaminant of 123I is:
   A. 124I
   B. 122I
   C. stannous chloride
   D. alumina

A. is correct.
Caution is advised when using 123I prepared by the $p, 2n$ method because of the 124I contaminant.

5.051 Radioaerosol particle sizing must be within the following range:
   A. 0.25 - 1.00 u
   B. 0.50 - 3.00 u
   C. 5.00 - 10.00 u
   D. 10.00 -15.00 u

B. is correct.
Particles in the range of .5u to 3.0u can reach the alveoli and be deposited there. Larger particles (10 to 15 u) are filtered out of the system through the delivery system.
Smaller particles may escape through expiration.

5.052 ^{99m}Tc-hexamethyl propylamineoxime (HMPAO) is a lipophilic brain agent also known as:
   A. ^{99m}Tc DTPA
   B. Cardiolite
   C. ^{99m}Tc-exametazime
   D. Macrotec
   E. Neurolite

C. is correct.

5.053 Which of the following functions of the liver is utilized in imaging the liver using an "IDA" compound?
  A. bile production and secretion
  B. vitamin and mineral storage
  C. fat metabolism
  D. particulate phagocytosis

A. is correct.
The "IDA" compounds, used for hepatobiliary imaging, are removed from the blood by the same processes that transport and excrete bilirubin and are specific to the functioning hepatocytes in the liver.

5.054 The majority of radiolabeled particles used for pulmonary perfusion imaging should fall within the range:
  A. below 1 u
  B. 1 to 10 u
  C. 15 to 70 u
  D. 70 to 100 u

C. is correct.
Distribution of particles for perfusion imaging is based on pulmonary blood flow. The smallest vessels in the lungs range from approximately 7 to 10 um in diameter and will easily trap particles larger than 10 um. This mechanism of localization is called capillary blockade.

5.055 The principle radionuclide contaminant of a ^{99m}Tc eluant is:
  A. alumina ion
  B. molybdenum
  C. pyrogens
  D. free pertechnatate

B. is correct.
A radionuclidic contaminant is defined as the proportion of the total radioactivity that is not present as the stated radionuclide. (as the presence of ^{99}Mo in the ^{99m}Tc eluent)

5.056 Which of the following best describes Xenon 133 gas?
  A. 25 keV alpha emitter
  B. 80 keV beta-gamma emitter
  C. 140 keV beta-gamma emitter
  D. 70 keV beta emitter

B. is correct.
133Xe has a 80 keV gamma plus significant beta emissions and so is considered a beta-gamma emitter.

5.057 Which of the following radiopharmaceuticals will best evaluate the renal cortex?
  A. ^{99m}Tc DTPA
  B. ^{99m}Tc DMSA
  C. ^{99m}Tc GH
  D. 131I hippuran

B. is correct.
DMSA concentrates in the renal cortex (approximately 42% at 6 hours) and is used when cortical detail is important.

5.058 Instant thin layer chromatography for water - insoluble radiopharmaceuticals reveals:
  A. percent binding
  B. reduced hydrolyzed
  C. free ^{99m}Tc
  D. radionuclide purity

C. is correct.
For water-insoluble radiopharmaceuticals, it is not possible to separate the reduced hydrolyzed using this rapid system. The free pertechnatate can be determined.

5.059 Reoxidation of ^{99m}Tc may be reduced by packaging the nonradioactive reagent kit in:
  A. an oxygen atmosphere
  B. a nitrogen atmosphere
  C. a hydrogen atmosphere
  D. a moisture-free atmosphere

B. is correct.
The presence of oxygen in reagent kits will degrade the ^{99m}Tc-pharmaceutical complex.

5.060 When testing MAA and using acetone as an ITLC solvent, free ^{99m}Tc is evident at the:
  A. solvent front
  B. relative front
  C. origin
  D. centerpoint

A. is correct.
Free ^{99m}Tc04- can be measured at the solvent front or Rf = 1.

5.061 Commonly used ITLC solvents include:
1. acetone
2. methyl ethyl ketone
3. saline
A. 1 and 2
B. 1 and 3
C. 2 and 3
D. 1, 2, and 3

D. is correct.
Instant thin layer chromatography silica gel-impregnated strips are developed in solvents such as saline, acetone, and methyl ethyl ketone (MEK).

5.062 Solvents used during ITLC move via:
1. active transport
2. adsorption
3. capillary action
A. 1 and 2
B. 1 and 3
C. 2 and 3
D. 1, 2, and 3

C. is correct.
Chromatography takes advantage of the different velocities of the chemical components in the mobile phase and along a stationary phase (adsorbent).

5.063 An Iodine 123 capsule, contained in a glass vial, will result in a _____ when compared to a capsule contained in a plastic vial.
A. lower assay due to the attenuation of low-level photons
B. high assay due to contamination
C. significantly lower assay due to a photoelectric effect
D. much higher assay due to the volatility of iodine

A. is correct.
The glass vial having a higher density, will attenuate more of the low level photons than the plastic.

5.064 Particle size of ^{99m}Tc sulfur colloid preparations are affected by all of the following EXCEPT the:
A. amount of ^{99m}Tc added to the preparation
B. amount of gelatin used
C. heating time
D. presence of contaminants

A. is correct.
Particle size distribution can be affected by the amount of gelatin used, the heating time and the presence of contaminants such as aluminum cations. It is important to prepare the radiopharmaceutical in the same way each day so that particle size distribution does not create artifacts on the images.

SECTION 6: SKELETAL SCINTIGRAPHY

TUTORIAL

The skeleton is the framework of bone and cartilage that protects our internal organs and allows us to move by acting as levers for our muscles. In addition to support, protection, and movement, the bones store several minerals that can be supplied to the body on demand and in certain bones, the red marrow is capable of producing blood cells. The two parts of the skeleton are the axial skeleton (those structures along the central axis of the body) and the appendicular skeleton (pectoral and pelvic girdles and appendages).

Bone is one of the hardest materials in the body due to the inorganic salts deposited in its ground substance in an apatite crystal form, primarily calcium phosphate and calcium carbonate. Osteoblasts are cells responsible for forming new bone during growth and repair, while osteoclasts are responsible for the resorption of bone tissues. Bones replaces itself at different rates in various body regions throughout adult life. Remodeling allows old, disease, or injured bone to be removed and replaced with new bone tissue.

Skeletal scintigraphy takes advantage of the metabolic activity and vascularity of bone to produce images of diagnostic value to the clinician. It remains one of the most commonly ordered nuclear medicine studies. Clinical indications for bone scintigraphy include:

1. Tumor - primary or metastatic (detection, follow-up to therapy)

2. Infection - osteomyelitis vs cellulitus; septic arthritis

3. Trauma - especially occult fractures, stress fractures not demonstrated radiographically

4. Metabolic processes - arthritis, Padget's disease, endocrine disorders (hypothyroiditis, hypoparathyroidism), osteoporosis (bone densitometry)

5. Evaluation of bone pain

^{99m}Tc labeled phosphate compounds are used for bone imaging; ^{99m}Tc MDP (methylene diphosphonate) and ^{99m}Tc HDP (hydroxymethylene diphosphonate) with a blood clearance of 3 - 4 hours post administration, give comparable images and are both currently in use.

Patient preparation should include instructions to drink fluids and void frequently to clear the radiopharmaceutical from the body and reduce the dose to the bladder walls. Metal objects and prostheses should be removed prior to scanning to avoid attenuation artifacts. As with all studies, a patient history should be taken and correlation to the ordered exam evaluated.

In general, skeletal imaging is extremely sensitive and is most frequently used to evaluate and stage malignant carcinomas. Normal distribution of the radiopharmaceutical is symmetrical in the skeleton and activity in the kidneys and bladder is evidence of the urinary excretion of the radiopharmaceutical.

6.001 Which of the following functions does the skeleton perform?
   A. support
   B. protection
   C. mineral storage (especially calcium)
   D. site for blood cell formation
   E. B and C only
   F. all of the above

F. is correct.
Besides providing support and protection as internal framework, the skeleton provides a system of levers working with the muscular system to produce movement. Bones are metabolically active connective tissue storing many minerals (most importantly calcium) and red marrow cavities of bone provide a site for hematopoiesis or blood cell formation.

6.002 Included in the appendicular skeleton are:
   A. upper and lower extremities
   B. thoracic cage and sternum
   C. vertebral column
   D. pectoral and pelvic girdles
   E. A and D
   F. B and C

E. is correct.
While the appendicular skeleton consists of the bones of the limbs or appendages, the axial skeleton includes the skull, thoracic cage, vertebral column and sacrum (bones that lie around the body's center of gravity).

6.003 As osteoclastic activity increases in relationship to osteoblastic activity, bone deposition:
   A. increases
   B. decreases or ceases
   C. remains the same

B. is correct.
Osteoclasts are cells that destroy or resorb bone tissue, while osteoblasts are bone forming cells.

6.004 In a person who is 45 years old or older, bone resorption is _____ bone deposition.
   A. equal to
   B. greater than
   C. less than

B. is correct.
Two principal effects of aging on the skeletal system include the loss of calcium from the bones and a decreased ability to produce the organic portion of bone matrix.

6.005 Hydroxyapatite salts of the bone consist of:
   A. stannous pyrophosphate
   B. calcium, strontium, phosphorus
   C. phosphorus and hydroxide
   D. calcium phosphate and calcium carbonate
   E. all of the above

D. is correct.
Hydroxyapatites consist primarily of calcium phosphate $(Ca_3(PO_4)_2)$ and some calcium carbonate $(CaCO_3)$. The hydroxyapatites comprise approximately 67% of the bone weight.

6.006 Bone, once it is formed:
   A. remains stable throughout the normal life span
   B. undergoes alteration in disease states only
   C. undergoes change at the site of fracture or infection
   D. undergoes continuous change

D. is correct.
Bone is a metabolically active tissue exchanging nutrients in the blood supplying the bone tissue. Bone growth and remodeling are a part of the homeostasis of normal development.

6.007 The outer portion of all bones is covered by:
   A. periosteum
   B. articular cartilage
   C. compact bone
   D. endosteum
   F. spongy bone

A. is correct.
The periosteum is essential for bone growth and development. It also serves as a point of attachment for tendons and ligaments.

6.008 Bone loses _____ % of its calcium content before it is detectable on a ^{99m}Tc MDP (or HDP) bone scan.
   A a minimal
   B 20
   C 30
   D 50

A. is correct.
This is a factor in the sensitivity of bone imaging.

6.009 Bone loses_____ % of its calcium content before a lesion is detectable on a plain radiograph.
   A. a minimal - 5
   B. 10 - 20
   C. 30 - 50
   D. 50 - 70

C. is correct.
30 - 50 % decalcification of the bone is necessary to detect a bone lesion radiographically.

6.010 The mechanism by which ^{99m}Tc labeled compounds accumulate in the bone is:
   A. ionic exchange
   B. active transport
   C. compartmental localization
   D. Capillary blockade

A. is correct.
Radio-labeled bone agents are absorbed by the bone in a manner that reflects both the vascularity and local osteoblastic activity of the bone. Calcium analogs and phosphates will exchange with the non-labeled ions in the bone.

6.011 The organ receiving the greatest radiation dose using ^{99m}Tc phosphate bone imaging agent is:
   A. bones
   B. kidneys
   C. bone marrow
   D. bladder
   E. liver

D. is correct.
The dose to the bladder wall can be reduced by increasing fluid intake and frequent voiding.

6.012 The amount of soft tissue activity seen on a bone scan is related to:
   A. the tagging efficiency of the radiopharmaceutical
   B. the dose to scan time
   C. the age of the patient
   D. the patient's renal function
   E. all of the above
   F. A and B only

E. is correct.
Anything that will delay clearance of the radiopharmaceutical from the blood will increase the soft tissue activity seen during scanning.

6.013 Imaging of the skeleton with radiotracers is an important diagnostic tool because the skeleton is:
   A. a rare site of metastases from neoplasms which are primary elsewhere in the body
   B. a frequent site of metastases from neoplasms which are primary elsewhere
   C. a frequent site of primary neoplasms
   D. a site of bone marrow formation

B. is correct.
The skeleton is a frequent site of metastases from breast, prostate, lung and renal carcinomas.

6.014 In the ^{99m}Tc polyphosphate bone image, the inferior tips of the scapulae can easily be mistaken for:
   A. rib lesions
   B. xipoid lesion
   C. metastatic lung tumor
   D. breast lesions

A. is correct.
Having the patient raise his/her arms for imaging, or taking oblique views will help differentiate rib lesions from the scapular tips.

6.015 The usual adult dose for bone scintigraphy using ^{99m}Tc agents is:
   A. 2 - 3 mCi
   B. 4 - 7 mCi
   C. 10 - 15 mCi
   D. 15 - 20 mCi

D. is correct.
The adult dose is usually 20 mCi (740 MBq); the pediatric dose is based on weight.

6.016 Interpreting a bone scan as normal on the basis of symmetrical appearance of skeletal activity can be a drawback in which of the following conditions?
  A. osteosarcoma
  B. osteoarthritis
  C. osteomyelitis
  D. osteoid osteoma

B. is correct.
A degenerative joint disease, osteoarthritis is often seen bilaterally in the shoulders, knees, and other joints of the body.

6.017 Bone imaging is particularly useful in detecting metastases in areas which are difficult to visualize radiographically. These areas may include:
  A. the sternum
  B. the scapulae
  C. the thoracic vertebrae
  D. A and B only
  E. all of the above

E. is correct.
Because of the superimposition of overlying structures and anatomic location, these areas of the body are often difficult to image with conventional radiographs.

6.018 Radiographs provide fine structural detail of the skeleton, and:
  A. can visualize primary sites of bone malignancy
  B. can detect bone lesions earlier than bone imaging
  C. can detect metastatic lesions with a minimal change in bone density
  D. B and C only
  E none of the above

A. is correct.
Radiographs can demonstrate the sites of primary tumors and may be used to confirm the presence of metastatic disease evidenced on a bone scan.

6.019 Which of the following is the reason most frequently cited on a bone scan requisition?
  A. location and extent of primary bone tumor
  B. location and assessment of extent of metastatic bone lesions
  C. determination of the extent of arthritic disease
  D. evaluate osteomalacia

B. is correct.
Because of its sensitivity in detecting minimal bone changes, bone scintigraphy is the test of choice to locate and assess bone metastases.

6.020 Metastases usually present themselves in the _____ skeleton first.
  A. axial
  B. appendicular

A. is correct.
The vertebral column and ribs are often the first sites of bone metastases.

6.021 Bone cancers, metastases, and other bone disorders produce extremely high levels of _____ in the blood.
  A. lactic dehydrogenase
  B. alkaline phosphatase
  C. amylase
  D. creatinine kinase

B. is correct.
Increased blood levels of alkaline phosphate are an indication for bone scintigraphy.

6.022 Primary bone tumors are found most often in:
  A. children and young adults
  B. females
  C. the elderly
  D. A and B

A. is correct.
Ewings sarcoma, a malignant bone tumor is most prevalent in the first three decades of life.

6.023   A bone scan demonstrates an area of soft tissue uptake in the anterior region of the elbow. The most likely explanation for this activity is:
   A. soft tissue calcifications
   B. hyperactivity of osteoclasts in bone
   C. cellulitis
   D. extravasation of the bone scan dose

D. is correct.
A slight extravasation will demonstrate an increased area of activity at the site. The antecubital fossa is a common injection site and increased activity in this area should always be suspect for extravasation of the dose.

6.024   The principle of radionuclide bone scintigraphy is based on:
   A. the ability of diseased bone to hyperconcentrate the radiopharmaceutical
   B. the reparative response of bone to injury or destruction
   C. the similarity of the radiotracer to normal (native) bone constituents
   D. B and C

D. is correct.
The ion exchange of native and radiolabeled bone constituents and increased osteoblastic activity in response to injury, contribute to the formation of images in skeletal scintigraphy.

6.025   Which of the following may be considered a drawback encountered in radionuclide bone imaging?
   A. sensitivity to minimal bone changes
   B. nonspecificity of bone abnormalities
   C. uptake in the kidneys and bladder
   D. all of the above

B. is correct.
While very sensitive to bone abnormalities, bone scintigraphy is relatively non-specific in identifying bone lesions.

6.026   A pediatric bone scan should be compared to a "normal" pediatric bone scan rather than a "normal" adult bone scan because:
   A. there is increased uptake in the weight bearing areas of the axial skeleton of an older adult
   B. marked variations of regional turnover of bone seeking minerals occur at different ages
   C. there is increased uptake in the epipheseal plates of the pediatric patient
   D. all of the above
   E. A and C only

D. is correct.
It is advisable for each department to utilize examples of "normals" using their own radiopharmaceuticals, imaging device, and method of image recording and to match age and sex of the patient under evaluation to a similar "normal" example.

6.027   Normal renal function can be indicated on a bone scan by:
   A. equal kidney activity that is less than bone activity
   B. equal kidney activity that is significantly more intense than bone activity
   C. absence of kidney activity
   D. absence of bladder activity

A. is correct.
Phosphate labeled ^{99m}Tc agents are excreted through the urinary tract. Normal function will demonstrate bilateral kidney activity that is less than bone.

6.028   Visible rib lesions which are arranged in a linear fashion are generally indicative of:
   A. rib trauma
   B. rib metastases
   C. inflammation of the lungs
   D. all of the above

A. is correct.
Trauma to the ribs (especially after a fall) will appear as a straight line of lesions along the ribs.

6.029 Increased activity is noted in the lower cervical spine on a whole body bone scan performed on a seventy year old with no prior history of carcinoma. The activity is most likely to be due to:
  A. stress fracture
  B. degenerative changes
  C. Padgets disease
  D. thyroid gland activity
  E. osteomyelitis

B. is correct.
While overall skeletal activity in the elderly may be lower than in younger patients, arthritic, or degenerative changes are likely responsible for increased tracer concentration, especially in the spine, shoulders, knees, and other joints affected by arthritis.

6.030 A bone scan of a sixty year old man demonstrates a diffuse pattern of intensely increased activity in the skull, proximal femurs and one side of the pelvis. This appearance is typical of what disease process?
  A. Ewing's sarcoma
  B. Padget's disease
  C. multiple myeloma
  D. Legg-Perthe's disease
  E. renal failure

B. is correct.
Often there is so much uptake of the tracer in Padget's disease lesions that there is little uptake in the normal bone. The scan pattern is typical of Padget's lesions.

6.031 An intense "hot" spot appears to be overlying the soft tissue of the right thigh on the bone scan of a 2 year old with an initial diagnosis of osteomyelitis of the left ankle. What is the most probable cause of this activity?
  A. cellulitis of right thigh
  B. osteomyelitis of right thigh
  C. metastatic lesions from unidentified primary carcinoma
  D. urine contamination
  E. weight-bearing stress

D. is correct.
In a pediatric bone scan, unidentified intensely increased areas of activity that are not part of the osseous uptake, should be suspicious for urine contamination.

6.032 When performing three-phase bone imaging of the wrist, it is important to:
  A. position the right wrist in the center of the field of view
  B. use a pinhole collimator
  C. position both wrists in the field of view
  D. inject in the affected extremity

C. is correct.
Positioning both wrists in the field of view will give a relative comparison of the affected wrist to the contralateral side.

6.033 Of the choices given, the best dynamic acquisition parameters for a three-phase bone scan following the bolus intravenous injection of ^{99m}Tc MDP are:
  A. 10 serial images of 1 minute each
  B. 20 serial images of 3 seconds each
  C. 30 serial images of 1 second each
  D. 30 serial images of 60 seconds each

B. is correct.
This acquisition will give the best flow information in an appropriate amount of time.

6.034 Some disease states may be differentiated by obtaining early "blood-pool" images. Which of the following will show reduced tracer uptake in osseous tissue in delayed or repeated images?
  A. cellulitis
  B. osteoarthritis
  C. osteomyelitis
  D. recent fracture

A. is correct.
In cellulitis, a typical appearance on a three phase bone scan may demonstrate increased blood flow to the affected area, increased activity on the blood pool image with a "normal" osseous or bone uptake on delays. Acute osteomyelitis will have a focally abnormal (intense activity) on delayed static images.

6.035 Three phase bone imaging is beneficial except for which of the following:
   A. distinguishing chronic from acute osteomyelitis
   B. differentiating recent from old trauma
   C. diagnosing osteoporosis
   D. assessing differences in regional blood flow

C. is correct.
Osteoporosis results in reduction in the mass of bone.

6.036 The pattern of osteomyelitis in a three-phase bone scan would demonstrate:
   A. focal increased blood flow to the involved bone and diffuse activity of the tracer in the bone on delayed images
   B. diffuse increased blood flow to the involved bone and focal intense activity of tracer in the bone on delayed images
   C. diffuse increased blood flow to the involved bone and diffuse intense activity of the tracer in the bone on the delayed images
   D. focal increased blood flow to the involved bone and focal intense activity of the tracer in the bone on delayed images

D. is correct.
This is a typical appearance of osteomyelitis on a three-phase bone scan.

6.037 The usual route of administration of ^{99m}Tc pertechnatate for joint imaging is:
   A. intravenous
   B. intramuscular
   C. intrathecal
   D. intraperitoneal

A. is correct.
Images are acquired immediately after injection to assess increased areas of blood flow, as found with synovitis.

6.038 A bone scan is performed on a patient with metastatic colon cancer. The scan demonstrates focal soft tissue activity in the right upper quadrant. The most likely explanation for this activity is:
   A. soft tissue inflammation
   B. female breast activity
   C. liver metastases
   D. myocardial infarction

C. is correct.
The patient's history and the location of the lesion would direct the diagnostician to the finding of liver metastases. This could be confirmed with a sulfur colloid liver scan or CT (computed tomography).

6.039 All of the following are acceptable reasons for having a patient void before preforming a bone scan EXCEPT:
   A. imaging times may be extended because of the bladder activity
   B. excess activity in the bladder can obscure pelvic anatomy
   C. voiding reduces the dose to the bladder wall
   D. the patient will be more comfortable during the procedure

A. is correct.
The activity in the bladder may reduce imaging time in static imaging of the pelvis since the majority of the counts would be coming from the bladder rather than the bones.

6.040 Decreased tracer accumulation may be found in all of the following disease processes EXCEPT:
   A. bone cyst
   B. avascular necrosis
   C. arthritis
   D. multiple myeloma
   E. bone infarction

C. is correct.
In all forms of arthritis, there is an increase in the bone tracer adjacent to the affected joint.

6.041 Obtaining a patient history prior to bone scanning is relevant for all of the following EXCEPT:
   A. previous history of trauma
   B. previous radiation or chemotherapy
   C. medications the patient is currently taking
   D. location of pain patient is experiencing
   E. A and D only
   F. all can be relevant considerations

F. is correct.
Because of the sensitivity of bone scan imaging, anything that will affect the distribution of tracer in the body should be a considered relevant patient history.

6.042 If a shoulder or hip appears to have increased uptake not relevant to the the patient's history or complaint, the technologists first concern should be to:
   A. alert the attending physician to the problem
   B. ask the patient to roll on their side
   C. take oblique images of the affected area
   D. insure that the patient is lying flat and that the camera head is not angled

D. is correct.
Improper positioning of the patient or camera can result in appearance of increased tracer on one side relative to the other.

6.043 A patient with a known history of prostate cancer has a scan with intense osseous uptake and faint or absent renal activity. This is commonly known as:
   A. renal insufficiency
   B. multiple myeloma
   C. superscan
   D. patient-induced artifacts
   E. normal

C. is correct.
In advanced metastatic disease, the uptake in the metastatic lesions may be so intense, as to leave little tracer left for renal excretion. The absence of kidneys or bladder on a bone scan should be highly suspect of advanced metastatic disease. This is characteristic of a "superscan".

6.044 Bone scan may be read as negative (normal) in pure osteolytic bone disease.
   A. true
   B. false

A. is correct.
Bone images may be negative in purely osteolytic eosinophilic granuloma and multiple myeloma.

6.045 67Ga citrate and 111In-labeled leukocyte imaging may be used in conjunction with ^{99m}Tc diphosphonate imaging to detect osteomyelitis.
   A. true
   B. false

A. is correct.
Because of the lack of specificity of bone imaging, these studies may better detect active osteomyelitis and detect deep soft tissue infection.

6.046 Some patients with septic arthritis or osteomyelitis may have normal bone scans with ^{99m}Tc-labeled compounds, but abnormal 67Ga citrate images.
   A. true
   B. false

A. is correct.
67Ga is often used in conjunction with bone imaging to better define active inflammatory processes such as osteomyelitis.

6.047 Bone density measurements may be assessed by which of the following techniques?
   A. single-photon absorptiometry
   B. dual energy absorptiometry
   C. quantitative computed tomography
   D. all of the above

D. is correct.
While the quantitative computed tomography dual energy systems are more accurate, x-ray exposure is significantly increased over dual energy absoptiometry.

6.048 For bone density measurements in pediatric patients, the procedure preferred is:
   A. single-photon absorptiometry
   B. dual energy absorptiometry
   C. quantitative computed tomography
   D. all of the above

A. is correct.

SPA or single-photon absorptiometry should be the procedure of choice because of the low radiation dose from the 125I (~29 keV) and the fact that the long bones are undergoing the greatest change in bone growth. Older patients would undergo dual energy (photon) absorpiometry (DPA) or quantitative computed tomography (QCT).

SECTION 7: CARDIOVASCULAR SCINTIGRAPHY

TUTORIAL

The average adult heart is approximately 14 centimeters long and 9 centimeters wide and is located within the mediastinum of the thorax. The lungs form the lateral border, the thoracic spine the posterior border, and the sternum the anterior border. There are four chambers of the heart, the right and left atria, which receive blood returning to the heart and the right and left ventricles, which force the blood out of the heart into arteries. The flow of blood through the heart is as follows: blood that is relatively low in oxygen concentration from systemic circulation enters the right atrium through the vena cava; as the right atrium contracts, the blood is moved into the right ventricle through the tricuspid valve. The contraction of the right ventricle forces blood through the pulmonary valve into the pulmonary trunk and pulmonary arteries where it travels to the lungs to become oxygenated. From the lungs, the oxygenated blood returns to the left atrium of the heart via the pulmonary veins, enters the left ventricle through the bicuspid valve, and as the left ventricle contracts, the blood is forced through the aortic valve into the aorta and the systemic circulatory system. The first two branches of the aorta, the right and left coronary arteries, supply the tissues of the heart with oxygenated blood.

The cardiac cycle, conduction system, and the regulation of the cardiac cycle are controlled by parasympathetic and sympathetic nerve fibers. The electrocardiogram (ECG) records the electrical activity in the myocardium and can be used as a physiological trigger for studies that are conducted in nuclear medicine to examine the function of the heart.

Imaging of the heart in nuclear medicine can be divided into studies that examine the myocardium and studies that examine cardiac function. Myocardial imaging to detect and localize myocardial infarction sites can be accomplished with ^{99m}Tc pyrophosphate, which localizes in infarcted tissue. The mechanism of localization is believed to be through the calcium crystal formation that occurs in the dying myocardial tissue. Increased uptake in the region of the myocardium is an indication of an abnormal study.

Myocardial perfusion imaging to detect and localize myocardial ischemia utilizes 201Tl thallous chloride, a radiopharmaceutical that localizes in the muscles of the body in a manner similar to the uptake of potassium. Since the thallium will not localize in areas of infarcted tissue, it can be used to distinguish myocardial ischemia from infarction. Two ^{99m}Tc -labeled agents, ^{99m}Tc teboroximine (Cardio Tec, Squibb Diagnostics) and ^{99m}Tc sestimibi (Cardiolite, Du Pont Pharma) are also in use to evaluate myocardial perfusion. All three agents behave differently in the body and have their own imaging protocols. The studies are usually conducted during exercise (stress) and rest (redistribution). If a patient is unable to exercise due to physical disability, pharmacological stress agents such as dipyridamole may be used to increase coronary blood flow in a manner that is similar to exercise stress.

Cardiac functional imaging quantitatively evaluates such pumping abilities of the heart as; ejection fraction, stroke volume, and cardiac output. In addition, wall motion abnormalities can also be evaluated. Use of the first pass method using ^{99m}Tc pertechnatate or ^{99m}Tc DTPA is often referred to as radionuclide angiography since the material passes through the heart one chamber at a time and evaluation of right ventricular ejection fraction can be more accurately accomplished.

The gated blood pool method or radionuclide ventriculogram most often is used to examine the function of the left ventricle. Red blood cells are labeled with ^{99m}Tc using an in vivo, in-vitro, or modified in vivo - in vitro technique. Acquisitions may be performed at rest or during exercise and are acquired using the R wave of the patients' ECG as a physiologic trigger to acquire images over the cardiac cycle. This allows for calculation of the ejection fraction from the region drawn over the left ventricle and viewing of the "cine" image to evaluate wall motion abnormalities such as dyskinesis, akinesis, hypokinesis, or aneurysms.

Nuclear cardiology has become an extremely important part of the nuclear medicine department and is establishing its validity as a screening modality for more invasive diagnostic techniques.

7.001 The heart is located in the center of the chest, directly above the diaphragm, just beneath the sternum in a space between the lungs called the:
    A. pericardium
    B. precordium
    C. mediastinum
    D. peritoneum

C. is correct.
The heart is located in the middle mediastinum and is partially covered by the lungs.

7.002 The circulation that carries oxygenated blood from the left ventricle of the heart to body tissues is called the _____ circulation.
    A. pulmonic
    B. systemic
    C. regulatory
    D. systolic

B. is correct.
The distribution of oxygenated blood to the body's tissues begins at the left side of the heart.

7.003 The coronary artery circulation receives approximately _____% of the cardiac output of the heart.
    A. 4-5
    B. 10
    C. 20
    D. 25

A. is correct.
The continuous activity of the heart requires a constant supply of oxygen. The coronary arteries carry the oxygenated blood from the aorta to the heart muscle.
Some sources state that the myocardium receives as much as 10% of the cardiac output.

7.004 Venous blood from the body is delivered to the _____ chamber of the heart.
    A. left atrium
    B. left ventricle
    C. right atrium
    D. right ventricle

C. is correct.
The thin walled right atrium receives blood from the superior and inferior vena cava before passing through the tricuspid valve into the right ventricle.

7.005 Oxygenated blood is returned to the heart by the _____ which enter the left side of the heart.
    A. aorta
    B. pulmonary veins
    C. coronary arteries
    D. pulmonary artery

B. is correct.
Oxygenated blood enters the left atrium through the pulmonary veins, then passes through the mitral valve during ventricular diastole.

7.006 Which is the best view to delineate the left ventricle on a nuclear medicine scan?
    A. left lateral
    B. left posterior oblique
    C. anterior
    D. left anterior oblique (45-60%)
    E. right anterior oblique (45-60%)

D. is correct.
The left anterior oblique is generally the best view to separate the left ventricle from the right ventricle. The exact angle should be optimized for each patient.

7.007 The electrocardiogram (ECG) presents a visible record of the heart's:
  A. output
  B. left ventricular ejection fraction
  C. contraction
  D. wall motion
  E. electrical activity

E. is correct.
The heart's electrical activity is demonstrated on the ECG which has been used as a diagnostic test for the heart's conduction system for over 85 years.

7.008 The left ventricle of the heart (in the "normal" patient) holds approximately _____mls of blood during end diastole.
  A. 50
  B. 75
  C. 100
  D. 150

D. is correct.
This quantity of blood is called the end-diastolic volume.

7.009 The stroke volume of the left ventricle is:
  A. the volume of blood that remains in the ventricle per beat
  B. the difference between end diastolic and systolic volumes
  C. the ejection fraction
  D. the difference between cardiac output and blood pressure measurements

B. is correct.
Stroke volume is defined as the amount of blood pumped by the left ventricle into the aorta with each beat. SV = EDV -ESV

7.010 The status of the ventricles when in end diastole is:
  A. they are at peak emptying
  B. they are at peak filling
  C. they are represented by the T-wave on the ECG
  D. an abnormal ECG characteristic

B. is correct.
Cardiac diastole represents the a period of relaxation, when the ventricles fill with blood.

7.011 The thick muscular wall that separates the right and left ventricles is called:
  A. posterior wall
  B. interventicular septum
  C. inferior wall
  D. antero-lateral wall

B. is correct.
Because the systemic arteries carry blood at a higher pressure than the pulmonary arteries, the left ventricular walls are thicker than the right.

7.012 A graphic representation of the depolarization and repolarization of heart muscle and sensed by electrodes placed on the body's surface is called:
  A. an action potential curve
  B. the cardiac cycle
  C. an electrocardiogram
  D. a precordial lead

C. is correct.
The ECG records the variations in voltage produced by the heart during the different phases of the cardiac cycle.

7.013 A normal heart beat is:
  A. arrythmic
  B. synchronic
  C. bradycardiogenic
  D. cyanotic
  E. anoxic

B. is correct.
Synchrony is a characteristic of the healthy heart where the entire myocardium contracts more or less simultaneously.

7.014 The QRS complex represents the:
   A. depolarization of the ventricles
   B. repolarization of the ventricles
   C. the resting state of the ventricles
   D. the beginning of the SA-node stimulation

A. is correct.
The QRS complex consists of an initial downward deflection (Q wave), a large upward deflection (R wave), and a second downward deflection (S wave). These waves represent the time it takes for the impulse to complete ventricular activation.

7.015 The electrical conduction in the heart originates by initiation of impulses in the:
   A. Purkinge fiber system
   B. AV node
   C. Bundle of His
   D. SA node

D. is correct.
The sinoatrial node (SA node) is the heart's pacemaker, initiating impulses automatically.

7.016 The sympathetic nervous system is responsible for:
   A. increasing the permeability of the myocardium to potassium
   B. decreasing heart rate and cardiac output
   C. increasing the heart rate by increasing the permeability of sodium into the cardiac cell
   D. all of the above

C. is correct.
The resting potential is stimulated, depolarization takes place, and repolarization begins. This series of events is responsible for the contraction of the myocardium.

7.017 The "normal" resting heart rate is:
   A. bradycardic
   B. tachycardic
   C. 60 - 100 beats per minute
   D. 100 -120 beats per minute
   E. asystolic

C. is correct.
Depending upon age, gender, physical condition and physical activity, the average resting heart rate is between 60 - 100 beats per minute.

7.018 The volume of blood pumped by the left ventricle per unit time is known as the:
   A. cardiac volume
   B. cardiac output
   C. ejection fraction
   D. stroke volume

B. is correct.
Cardiac output by definition, is the volume of blood discharged from the left or right ventricle per minute. For the average adult at rest, cardiac output is approximately 3.0 liters per square meter of body surface per minute. The stroke volume x the heart rate determines the cardiac output.

7.019 The myocardial muscle mass tapers as it approaches the apex.
   A. true
   B. false

A. is correct.
The wall of the apex is usually the thinnest part of the left ventricle and can be seen on nuclear medicine images as a decrease in activity.

7.020 The best imaging period for the evaluation of acute myocardial infarcts with ^{99m}Tc pyrophosphate is _____ post infarction.
   A. 0 -24 hours
   B. 24 -72 hours
   C. 1 - 5 days
   D. 5 - 7 days

B. is correct.
The time of maximum deposition of pyrophosphate is usually 48 - 72 hours after infarction.

7.021 A major disadvantage of ^{99m}Tc-PYP imaging is:
   A. the radiation dose to the patient
   B. the insensitivity of the test to distinguish between infarct and ischemia
   C. patient cardiac motion
   D. the delay between imaging and onset of symptoms

D. is correct.
Since the time for maximum deposition of pyrophosphate is 48 - 72 hours after infarction, the indications for the exam would be more likely to include defining the areas of infarction than in diagnosing an infarction.

7.022 The mechanism of localization of ^{99m}Tc PYP in the necrosed myocardial tissue is best explained by:
  A. the deposition of potassium in the damaged myocardial cell
  B. the deposition of calcium in the damaged myocardium
  C. mitochondrial accumulation of denatured proteins
  D. all of the above
  E. none of the above

B. is correct.
The accumulation of calcium within the mitochondria and within the cytoplasm of necrotic cells of a myocardial infarction correlate with the sites of maximum pyrophosphate accumulation.

7.023 A ^{99m}Tc pyrophosphate scan would require all of the following for the best scan results EXCEPT:
  A. high resolution collimator
  B. 500 - 1000K counts per planar image
  C. a 2 - 3 hour post injection delay prior to planar imaging
  D. treadmill testing using the "Bruce" protocol

D. is correct.
Exercise would not affect the myocardial uptake in infarcted tissue.

7.024 Persistent diffuse activity in the myocardium region noted on pyrophosphate imaging at 1 - 2 hours post injection may indicate:
  A. the need for 48 hour delayed views
  B. the need for further delayed imaging
  C. blood pool activity in the myocardium
  D. A and C only
  E. B and C only

E. is correct.
Images recorded between 4 - 6 hours post injection minimize the possibility of blood pool activity which may be mistaken for diffuse myocardium uptake.

7.025 Occasionally, an extensive transmural infarct may present itself as a large area of increased tracer activity (on a pyrophosphate scan) with a central zone of relatively decreased intensity. This is called the:
  A. pericardial effusion
  B. pericarditis
  C. unstable angina
  D. the doughnut sign
  E. the half-moon sign

D. is correct.
The doughnut sign (a ring of activity surrounding large anterior wall infarcts) usually indicates a poor prognosis.

7.026 The typical dose for a ^{99m}Tc pyrophosphate scan is:
  A. 1 - 5 mCi
  B. 5 - 10 mCi
  C. 15 - 20 mCi
  D. 20 - 25 mCi

C. is correct.
The usual dose of ^{99m}Tc pyrophosphate is 15 - 20 mCi (555 - 740 MBq) .

7.027 The maximum heart rate for an individual may be calculated by:
  A. 75% of the stroke volume
  B. an ejection fraction of 50 - 60 %
  C. 220 - patient's age
  D. cardiac output - stroke volume

C. is correct.
The predicted maximum heart rate per age is calculated as 220 - patient's age in years.

7.028 Which of the following radiopharmaceuticals is not used to perform myocardial perfusion imaging?
  A. ^{99m}Tc sestimibi
  B. ^{99m}Tc teboroxime
  C. 111In oxine
  D. 201Tl Cl

C. is correct.
Myocardial perfusion imaging is usually performed using 201Tl as thallous chloride or one of the ^{99m}Tc based agents.

7.029 A maximal exercise test indicates attainment of:
  A. 50 - 70 % of the maximum heart rate
  B. 85 - 100 % of the maximum heart rate
  C. chest pain by the patient
  D. drop in patients blood pressure during exercise

B. is correct.

7.030 The usual time delay for the redistribution images post 201Tl exercise imaging is:
  A. 20 minutes
  B. 90 minutes
  C. 2 - 4 hours
  D. 24 hours
  E. 1 week

C. is correct.
The 4 hour redistribution imaging may underestimate the extent of viable myocardium. Late imaging at 24 - 72 hours with reinjection has demonstrated redistribution of 201 Tl that appeared irreversible at 2 - 4 hours.

7.031 A fixed defect noted on a two-injection 201Tl study would most likely reflect:
  A. normal myocardium
  B. ischemic myocardium
  C. infarcted myocardium
  D. breast artifact commonly seen in males

C. is correct.
A persistent defect would most likely represent myocardial scarring from a myocardial infarction.

7.032 If a reversible defect is seen in the antero-septal and septal walls during 201Tl scintigraphy, it is most likely due to:
  A. an occluded left circumflex artery
  B. a narrowed left anterior descending artery
  C. a narrowed right coronary artery
  D. an occluded left anterior descending artery

B. is correct.
Stress induced defects which reverse or normalize in redistribution images most likely represent myocardial ischemia rather than an occlusion.

7.033 The presence of excessive 201Tl activity (greater than 50% lung:heart) in the lungs has consistently been demonstrated to be:
  A. a sign of tricuspid valve disease
  B. a sign of left ventricular dysfunction
  C. a characteristic of right to left shunts
  D. evidence for bypass surgery

B. is correct.
Increased thallium uptake in the lungs usually signifies multivessel disease and left ventricular dysfunction due to prolonged pulmonary transit time and increased left atrial pressure.

7.034 Causes for a false negative thallium study would include all of the following EXCEPT:
  A. patient was not exercised adequately
  B. the patient had no complaint of chest pain during the study
  C. planar imaging was performed more than 30 minutes after injection of tracer
  D. there was a global decrease in tracer throughout the myocardium noted in patients with three vessel disease

B. is correct.
A complaint of chest pain during a thallium study may be reason to terminate the stress test; absence of pain would not be the cause of a false negative study.

7.035 Beta-blockers and digitalis will _____ 201 Tl uptake in the myocardium.
  A. increase
  B. decrease
  C. have no effect on

B. is correct.
Drugs that affect the response to and interpretation of exercise tests should be discontinued prior to testing under the direct order of the physician.

7.036 Dipyridamole is mainly used as an intervention in 201Tl scintigraphy to:
   A. evaluate abnormal treadmill patients
   B. investigate CAD (coronary artery disease) in patients who cannot tolerate treadmill exercise protocols
   C. improve the quality of 201Tl uptake in the heart
   D. evaluate patients with valvular disease

B. is correct.
Pharmacologic stress testing (using an agent such as dipyridamole) is an alternative to exercise stress testing when a patient may be limited by cardiovascular, pulmonary, or peripheral vascular disease.

7.037 Soft tissue attenuation (such as breast artifact) may lead to:
   A. false negative 201Tl studies
   B. false positive 201Tl studies
   C. improvement in the detection of coronary artery stenosis
   D. require a repeat treadmill study

B. is correct.
Breast artifacts may appear as a circular "cold defect" along the left ventricular anterior wall. To avoid breast artifacts on 201Tl images on female patients, some sites tape the breast above the mediastinum during imaging.

7.038 In dipyridamole testing, the use of low-level exercise after the administration of the dipryridamole would:
   A. increase the heart rate and diminish scan quality
   B. require aminophylline injections
   C. reduce non-cardiac side effects of the Persantine
   D. allow the cardiologist to study the patient further

C. is correct.
Patients injected during even minimal exercise have images of better contrast and have fewer side effects than those injected at rest.

7.039 The injection of dipyridamole is administered into the patient intravenously and within _____ minutes to ensure maximum saturation levels in the blood.
   A. 2
   B. 4
   C. 10
   D. 20

B. is correct.
A controlled infusion method is recommended.

7.040 Dipyridamole -thallium studies are done on patients with:
   A. physical limitations
   B. neurologic impairment
   C. non-diagnostic 201 Tl treadmill tests
   D. all of the above

D. is correct.
Pharmacologic stress testing using an agent such as dipyridamole offers an alternative to exercise stress testing in patients for whom exercise thallium may not be possible or appropriate.

7.041 Dipyridamole given intravenously or in large oral doses produces a vasodiliatory effect in both the epicardial and endocardial vessels, thereby:
   A. increasing the coronary flow
   B. increasing the interstitial adenosine levels
   C. increasing the 201 Tl uptake
   D. all of the above

D. is correct.
When used in addition to thallium imaging to assess myocardial perfusion, dipyridamole increases coronary blood flow and elevates intravascular adenosine levels thereby increasing the uptake of 201 Tl.

7.042 Concentration of 201 Tl is indirectly related to blood flow.
   A. true
   B. false

B. is correct.
201 Tl is concentrated in stressed muscle in direct dependence to the availability of blood vessels to carry the dose to muscle cells. Anything that disrupts the blood flow will interfere with the uptake of thallium in that region.

7.043 The patient preparation for dipyridamole 201Tl studies is (are):
   A. NPO 4 - 6 hours prior
   B. no caffeine or coffee within a minimum of 4 - 6 hours of the test
   C. no theophylline compounds within 48 hours of the test
   D. all of the above

D. is correct.
Some drugs have shown to have an antagonistic effect on the action of IV dipyridamole and a non-diagnostic study may result. Discontinuance of theophylline is a clinical judgment based on the patient's condition and history.

7.044 A second injection given at rest as a part of a 201Tl exercise/rest examination will:
   A. evaluate a fixed myocardial perfusion defect properly
   B. reveal the same information as the redistribution images
   C. increase the rate of false positive scan findings
   D. degrade image quality by flooding the blood with more tracer

A. is correct.
Viable myocardium will be "unmasked" using a second injection. Fixed or irreversible defects will be unaffected.

7.045 The rate of administration for intravenous dipyridamole is:
   A. 0.0142 mg/kg/min
   B. 0.142 mg/kg/sec
   C. 0.0142 mg/kg/sec
   D. 0.142 mg/kg/min

D. is correct.

7.046 Areas of the myocardium supplied by stenotic vessels will have less 201 Tl uptake due to a decreased blood flow and a slower 201 Tl intrinsic washout.
   A. true
   B. false

A. is correct.
There is a direct relationship between the blood flow in a given area and the uptake of thallium.

7.047 A subendocardial MI is reflective of necrosis throughout the myocardial wall.
   A. true
   B. false

B. is correct.
A subendocardial infarction involves only the layer of muscle beneath the endocardium. It does not involve the entire thickness of the myocardial wall.

7.048 Dipyridamole is contraindicated in evaluation of patients with the following
   A. known brochospastic lung disease
   B. systemic hypotension
   C. unstable angina
   D. acute MI
   E. all of the above

E. is correct.

7.049 Common side effects of dipyridamole are:
   A. light headedness
   B. nausea
   C. flushing
   D. headache
   E. all of the above

E. is correct.
As with all pharmacologic stress agents, dipyridamole should be administered by the supervising physician or other qualified persons licensed to administer intravenous drugs and the patient observed for side effects.

7.050 Aminophylline-like compounds taken by the patient prior to 201Tl Persantine testing will:
   A. enhance 201Tl uptake in the myocardium
   B. depreciate the interventional effect of Persantine
   C. create immediate onset of observed adverse reactions
   D. depress the heart rate and blood pressure response

B. is correct.
Intravenous aminophylline has been shown to reverse the pharmacologic effects of IV Persantine (dipyrimadole) and similar compounds will counteract the effects of the dipyrimadole.

7.051 If a patient weighs 170 pounds and the persantine administered dose is 0.56 mg/kg of body weight. The patient would receive _____ milligrams of persantine.
   A. 25
   B. 37
   C. 43
   D. 52

C. is correct.
170 lbs = 77 kgs
77 kgs x .56 mg/kg = 43 mg

7.052 Based on the information in the previous question, the persantine ampules are 10mg/2mls. What volume (in mls) would be administered to this patient?
   A. 5.4
   B. 6.7
   C. 8.6
   D. 10.2

C. is correct.
10 mg / 2 ml = 5 mg / ml
43 mg / 5mg /ml = 8.6 ml

7.053 In a gated cardiac scan, the patient's heart rate is 60 beats per minute. If each cardiac cycle is divided into 20 equal time segments, the average time will be ____milliseconds long.
   A. .05
   B. 0.5
   C. 5.0
   D. 50

D. is correct.
The time for each image would be given by:
$$\frac{60sec}{heart\ rate\ x\ \#\ images} = \frac{60}{60\ x\ 20} = \frac{60}{1200} = .05\ sec$$

.05 seconds x $\frac{1000ms}{second}$ = 50 milliseconds

7.054 The physiologic trigger used as a gating signal in a RVG cardiac study is:
   A. respiration rate
   B. the p-wave
   C. the R-wave
   D. the technologist performing the study

C. is correct.

7.055 On a 45 degree LAO view on a RVG, a slight caudal tilt better separates the ventricles from:
   A. the atria
   B. the lungs
   C. each other
   D. the great vessels

A. is correct.
Slightly angling the camera head toward the feet will give better separation of the atria and ventricles.

7.056 Stroke volume ratios on a RVG study (L/R or R/L) can be biased by:
   A. improper position of the gated blood pool image
   B. the "halo effect"
   C. ischemia
   D. asymmetric peak imaging

A. is correct.
The blood pool image should have good separation of the ventricles.

7.057 The formula used for the calculation of the ejection fraction using end diastolic and end systolic counts of either ventricle is EF=:
    A. EDC+ ESC/EDC
    B. EDC - ESC/ESC
    C. EDC - ESC/ EDC - BKG
    D. ESC - EDC/BKG

C. is correct.
Ejection fraction can also be defined as:
stroke volume (EDV -ESV)
end diastolic volume

7.058 The RBC label commonly used in RVG (radionuclide ventriculogram) imaging may be affected by:
    A. a patient with a low hematocrit
    B. anticoagulants in the patient
    C. antiinflammatory agents
    D. all of the above
    E. B and C only

D. is correct.
Patient factors have been shown to affect RBC labeling.

7.059 Which of the following views is least likely to be performed in a typical RVG study?
    A. anterior
    B. LAO
    C. left lateral
    D. posterior

D. is correct.
The anterior views of the heart demonstrate the best separation of the chambers; the left lateral view is used for wall motion information; the posterior view is the least valuable view for the heart lies posteriorly on the thoracic vertebra. Right sided images are not routinely done because of the increased distance to the camera face.

7.060 A patient's ejection fraction normally _____ during periods of exercise.
    A. increases
    B. decreases
    C. remains the same

A. is correct.
The ejection fraction, or amount of blood pumped from the ventricles, increases during periods of exercise.

7.061 Labeling RVGs by the in-vitro or modified in-vivo methods will require:
    A. a SnCl2 complex
    B. incubation of the cells in the labeling medium
    C. a heparinized labeling syringe
    D. all of the above
    E. A and B only

D. is correct.
The stannous complex is necessary for the reduction of the pertechnatate; the incubation allows labeling of the RBCs; and the heparin is an anticoagulant to prevent the cells from clotting.

7.062 In the normal resting state, where coronary blood flow is relatively low with a high degree of peripheral vascular and coronary circulatory resistance, dipyridamole produces a:
    A. high flow, low resistance system
    B. high flow, high resistance system
    C. low flow, low resistance system
    D. low flow, high resistance system

A. is correct.
I.V. Dipyridamole increases coronary blood flow from 2 - 5 fold and acts primarily on smaller coronary vessels with a vasodilatory effect.

7.063 RVG evaluations are used for all of the following EXCEPT:
    A. evaluation pre and post CABG
    B. evaluation of CAD
    C. evaluation of LV and RV ejection fractions
    D. establishing the diagnosis of acute MI
    E. baseline testing of cardiac function prior to chemotherapy

D. is correct.
A, B, C, and E are all evaluations of the functional capabilities of the heart; a strength of RVG imaging.

7.064 A cine or playback tape of a RVG study may be used to determine the wall motion kinetics of the ventricles.
- A. true
- B. false

A. is correct.
An advantage of the radionuclide ventriculogram is the ability to put the images in cine mode to observe and evaluate wall motion.

7.065 The proper calculation of the computer assisted LVEFs is done by:
- A. analyzing the view which shows greatest RV to LV separation
- B. drawing ROIs that adhere closely to the ventricular volume
- C. making sure that the background ROI is not placed in a high activity area
- D. all of the above

D. is correct.
Inclusion of activity that does not reflect the ventricular counts will result in an inaccurate calculation of the ejection fraction.

7.066 In LVEF calculations, drawing a generous region of interest around the left ventricle or including part of the atrial areas would likely _____ the ejection fraction value.
- A. overestimate
- B. underestimate
- C. not affect

B. is correct.
Inclusion of activity outside the ventricle will falsely lower the ejection fraction.

7.067   Factors which affect cardiac ejection fraction determination include:
- A. ROI selection
- B. background ROI selection
- C. collimation used
- D. all of the above

D. is correct.
The ejection fraction is a quantitative determination of ventricular function and is affected by operator selection of ROIs and collimation. Distortions and inclusions of atria or major vessels will give a less accurate ejection fraction. Multicystal cameras give higher count density and better edge definition than the single crystal systems.

7.068 The right ventricle is difficult to evaluate for ejection fraction by this equilibrium method because:
- A. of overlying and underlying radioactive structures
- B. its often not analyzed in the proper view to create good separation between structures
- C. of its poor temporal resolution
- D. all of the above

D. is correct.
The first pass method to evaluate right ventricular ejection fractions is the test of choice.

7.069 The advantages of RVG over first pass studies is (are):
- A. multiple projections for a single dose administration
- B. better spatial resolution
- C. greater cardiac cycle sampling
- D. all of the above
- E. none of the above

D. is correct.
The development of cardiac radiopharmaceuticals that can be used for both first pass studies and radionuclide ventriculograms will allow information to be obtained from both studies with a single test.

7.070 Radioventriculograms are indicated for
- A. coronary artery perfusion disorders
- B. the evaluation of pulmonary emboli
- C. the quantification of ventricular function
- D. the recognition of cardiac arrhythmias

C. is correct.
The ejection fraction, which is the ratio of stroke volume (end-diastolic volume - end-systolic volume) to end-diastolic volume is a widely accepted measure of left ventricular function.

7.071 Which of the following is NOT consistent with the patient preparation for a resting RVG study?
  A. fasting
  B. electrodes are used for gating
  C. pre-tinning of RBCs
  D. a patient scan request

A. is correct.
Fasting is not required for a resting RVG.

7.072 The in-vivo labeling technique for gated blood pool imaging is preferred in some institutions due to:
  A. its increased labeling efficiency
  B. its increased technical difficulty
  C. its greater target to non-target ratio
  D. all of the above
  E. none of the above

E. is correct.
The in-vivo technique is technically easy to perform and has a labeling efficiency of approximately 90% compared to approximately 95% for the in-vitro method and greater than 95% for commercially prepared tagging agents.

7.073 The typical acquisition mode of RVGs is a collection in:
  A. 32 x 32 byte mode
  B. 64 x 64 word mode
  C. 128 x 128 mag mode
  D. 256 x 256 word mode

B. is correct.
A 64 x 64 word mode is a good compromise between image resolution and memory necessary to store the images. Word mode is preferred to byte mode because there is less chance of overwhelming the count limit per pixel with word mode.

7.074 In a typical RVG study, the suggested time that the tin complex should circulate in the body prior to pertechnetate injection is _____ minutes.
  A. 2-3
  B. 5-10
  C. 15-30
  D. >45

C. is correct.
The circulation for 15 to 30 minutes of the stannous pyrophosphate insures the bonding of the stannous ion to the red blood cells.

7.075 During an exercise RVG study a normal patient will demonstrate:
  A. decreased function of the heart with exercise
  B. increased ejection fraction by 5-10% from the resting calculations
  C. exercise protocol of 2 minutes per stage
  D. typical chest pain related to coronary disease

B. is correct.
The increase in ejection fraction during exercise is a normal function; some coronary disease results in reduced ejection fraction during exercise and evidence of wall motion abnormalities.

7.076 The most common computer collection mode of a resting RVG is:
  A. list mode
  B. dynamic list mode
  C. multi-gated frame mode
  D. word mode

C. is correct.
The resting RVG or gated equilibrium study collects data continuously over hundreds of cardiac cycles.

7.077 The functional images outputted in most RVG software programs best explains:
  A. wall motion abnormalities
  B. conduction abnormalities
  C. the presence of aneurysms
  D. all of the above

D. is correct.
The evaluation of the cine mode images provides information which are not obtained in the first-pass procedure.

7.078   The paradoxical functional image of a RVG is best identified as:
   A. arterial contraction
   B. aneurysmal ventricular motion
   C. hypokinetic areas of the myocardium
   D. all of the above

B. is correct.
The ventricles and atria are out of sync with one another. When the ventricles are in systole, the atria are in diastole.

7.079   A typical ^{99m}Tc labeled radiopharmaceutical dose for RVG imaging is:
   A. 1 -5 mCi
   B. 5 - 10 mCi
   C. 20 - 25 mCi
   D. 100 - 500 uCi

C. is correct.
The dose of 20 - 25 mCi (740 - 925 MBq) provides adequate counts for the equilibrium study.

7.080   A resting ejection fraction (LV) of 33% is considered:
   A. abnormal
   B. normal
   C. non-diagnostic
   D. dependent on department interpretation

A. is correct.
An ejection fraction below 50% would be considered abnormal. Many nuclear medicine laboratories use an average of 65% with a 5% deviation (55% - 75%).

7.081   The purpose of administering "cold" (unlabeled) PYP for red blood cell labeling with ^{99m}Tc is:
   A. to utilize the reducing agent in the pyrophosphate kit
   B. to cool the red blood cells to obtain maximum labeling efficiency
   C. to prevent clotting of the blood during the labeling process
   D. to increase the length of time that the label remains intact to allow for multiple views

A. is correct.
The stannous ion with bond with the red blood cells which allows the ^{99m}Tc to tag with the RBCs.

7.082   Persistent pulmonary activity and poor visualization of the left side of the heart represent _____ during a first pass evaluation.
   A. a ventricular aneurysm
   B. a left - to- right intracardiac shunt
   C. a right - to - left intracardiac shunt
   D. pulmonary hypertension

B. is correct.
The blood is shunted from the left side of the heart to the lungs.

7.083   If a patient developed worsening ST-segment depression during the exercise portion of a RVG study, the ejection fractions for the exercise study should show
   A. a pattern of continuous increase in EFs
   B. a pattern of lower ejection fractions during exercise
   C. an inability to attain a 5 - 10 % increase in EFs
   D. B and C only

D. is correct.
In the normal patient the ejection fraction will increase 5 - 10 % during exercise. Generally, the more severe the coronary disease, the lower the ejection fraction during exercise.

7.084   A multicrystal camera would be preferred to the conventional single crystal camera for performing first pass imaging because
   A. the images are more esthetically pleasing
   B. the detection of much higher count rates is possible
   C. great maneuverability of the imaging system

B. is correct.

SECTION 8: GENITOURINARY SCINTIGRAPHY

TUTORIAL

The primary function of the urinary system is to help keep the body in homeostasis and to regulate the volume and composition of extra cellular fluid which is accomplished through the formation of urine. The paired kidneys are located posteriorly, above the level of the waist. Of the two kidneys, the right kidney is slightly lower than the left because of the large area occupied by the liver. In addition to the two kidneys, the urinary tract is comprised of two ureters, the urinary bladder and the urethra. The kidneys receive approximately 25% of the total cardiac output through the right and left renal arteries.

The functional unit of the kidney is the nephron with other parts of the kidney serving primarily as storage areas or "tubes" to allow the passage of materials.

Nuclear medicine studies evaluate renal function, arterial and venous patency, glomerular filtration, tubular function, and urinary excretion. Because of their different modes of excretion, specific radionuclides may be used to evaluate certain elements of renal function.

Radionuclide	Dose	Function
^{99m}Tc DTPA	3-10mCi (111-370 MBq)	glomerular filtration
^{99m}Tc GH	10 mCi (370 MBq)	glomerular filtration; 5-10% tubular binding
^{99m}Tc DMSA	1-5 mCi (37-185 MBq)	glomerular filtration; 40-50% tubular binding
^{99m}Tc mertiatide (MAG3)	3-10 mCi (111-370 Mbq)	tubular secretion
131I hippuran	150-300uCi (5.55-11.1Mbq)	80-90% tubular secretion 10-20% filtration
123I hippuran	~250 uCi (9.25 Mbq)/kidney	same as for 131I hippuran

Radionuclide cystography and ureteral reflux studies are sensitive for even minute amounts of refluxed urine, especially in combination with computer enhanced acquisition and processing protocols. The typical study involves the instillation of 1-2 mCi of ^{99m}Tc pertechnatate into the urinary bladder via catheterization and dilution with sterile saline.

Testicular imaging to evaluate torsion of the testicle versus epididymitis is an important diagnosis since the therapy for torsion is surgery, while antibiotic therapy is prescribed for epididymitis. Doppler ultrasound is a non-invasive procedure to evaluate blood flow in the testes and is used in conjunction with, or in place of, radionuclide flow imaging to the testicles.

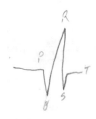

8.001 The vessel that carries blood to a cortical nephron is:
A. afferent arteriole
B. efferent arteriole
C. glomerulus
D. proximal convoluted tubule

A. is correct.
The afferent arteriole conducts blood from the renal artery to the glomerulus.

8.002 The functional unit of the kidney is the:
A. Bowman's capsule
B. calyx
C. loop of Henle
D. nephron

D. is correct.
The nephrons in the kidney function to produce urine.

8.003 The outer region of the kidneys is the:
A. calyx
B. cortex
C. medulla
D. pelvis

B. is correct.
The renal cortex contains the glomeruli and surrounds the calyces, medulla, and pelvis.

8.004 The loops of Henle descend into the:
A. calyx
B. cortex
C. medulla
D. pelvis

C. is correct.
The medulla is the inner region of the kidney and also contains the collecting ducts.

8.005 What is the correct order of passage from the plasma components in the nephron to the urine in the bladder?
        1. calyces and renal pelvis
        2. proximal convoluted tubule
        3. loop of Henle
        4. distal convoluted tubule
        5. Bowman's capsule
        6. ureter
A. 1, 2, 3, 4, 5, 6
B. 2, 1, 3, 4, 5, 6
C. 5, 2, 3, 4, 1, 6
D. 2, 3, 4, 1, 5, 6

C. is correct.
Represents the proper order for blood plasma components not needed by the body. Fluids that are not reabsorbed by the tubules are excreted as urine.

8.006 A normal adult glomerular filtration rate (GFR) is approximately:
A. 60 ml/min
B. 100 ml/min
C. 120 ml/min
D. 200 ml/min
E. 275 ml/min

C. is correct.
The 120 ml/min value is slightly higher in men than women.

8.007 The collecting ducts deposit urine into the:
A. calyces
B. cortex
C. medulla
D. pelvis

A. is correct.
The calyces then transport urine into the renal pelvis.

8.008 A normal adult excretes _____ mls of urine a day.
A. 500 - 1000
B. 1000 - 1500
C. 2000 - 2500
D. 2500 - 3000

B. is correct.
Although the amount may vary greatly depending on fluid intake, the minimum amount needed to rid the body of waste is 400 mls.

8.009   Diuretics can:
   A. increase blood pressure
   B. increase urine production
   C. decrease urine pressure
   D. stimulate ADH secretion

B. is correct.
Furosimide (Lassix) increases urine production and can also lower blood pressure.

8.010   Oliguria is:
   A. a bladder infection
   B. renal failure
   C. blood in urine
   D. renal insufficiency

D. is correct.
Oliguria is diminished urine production in relation to fluid intake (renal insufficiency).

8.011   The function of the kidney that helps to regulate blood pressure is:
   A. blood pH adjustment
   B. plasma volume control
   C. regulation of electrolyte concentrations
   D. secretion of prostaglandins

B. is correct.
The kidney performs all of these functions, but concentrating waste as urine changes the blood plasma volume. A decrease in plasma causes a decrease in blood pressure.

8.012   The most common malignant renal tumor in adults is:
   A. hypernephroma
   B. Wilm's tumor
   C. adenoma
   D. seminoma
   E. none of the above

A. is correct.
Hypernephromas are the most common malignant renal tumors. Wilm's tumors are malignant, but are most common in infants. Adenomas are benign.

8.013   It is best to locate kidney background regions for renogram curves:
   A. near the aorta
   B. near the kidneys
   C. near the lungs
   D. within the soft tissue in the pelvis
   E. none of the above

B. is correct.
Backgrounds need to mimic the tissue that would be left if the kidneys were not present.

8.014   Which agent would be preferred for SPECT imaging of the kidneys?
   A. 131 hippuran
   B. ^{99m}Tc MAG3
   C. ^{99m}Tc GH
   D. ^{99m}Tc DMSA

D. is correct.
^{99m}Tc DMSA collects in the tubular cells and provides good SPECT images of the kidneys once sufficient time (2-6 hours) is given for background activity to decrease.

8.015   Which pharmaceutical(s) provide delayed images of the kidneys?
   A. ^{99m}Tc DTPA
   B. ^{99m}Tc GH
   C. ^{99m}Tc DMSA
   D. A and B
   E. B and C
   F. A, B, and C

E. is correct.
^{99m}Tc GH and DMSA both accumulate in the tubular cells (cortices) and therefore can be imaged 2-6 hours after dosing.

8.016   Captopril renal scans are commonly ordered to evaluate:
   A. renal failure
   B. renal function
   C. renal hypertension
   D. GFR
   E. effective renal plasma flow (ERPF)

C. is correct.
Captopril renal scans are ordered to diagnose renal vascular hypertension (RVH) and renal artery stenosis (RAS).

8.017 Captopril is normally given _____ hours before the renal scan.
   A. .5
   B. 1
   C. 2
   D. 6
   E. 24

B. is correct.
The patient is given 50mg of Captopril orally before scanning and the patient's blood pressure is monitored closely thereafter.

8.018 A typical adult dose for ^{99m}Tc DTPA or 99mTc GH is:
   A. 100 - 150 uCi
   B. 5 -10 mCi
   C. 10 - 15 mCi
   D. 20 mCi

C. is correct.
The adult dose is 10 - 15 mCi, but pediatric doses are reduced by calculation or using a dose graph.

8.019 A typical dose for 131I hippuran is:
   A. 100-150 uCi
   B. 5 -10 mCi
   C. 10 - 15 mCi
   D. 20 mCi

A. is correct.
Pharmaceutical doses containing 131I are kept very small due to its higher energy (364kev) and the dose to the patient's thyroid from free 131I.

8.020 A typical dose for ^{99m}Tc DMSA is:
   A. 500 uCi
   B. 1 mCi
   C. 5 mCi
   D. 10 - 15 mCi
   E. 20 mCi

C. is correct.
This dose is lower than with ^{99m}Tc DTPA and ^{99m}Tc GH due to a higher dose of the radiopharmaceutical remaining in the kidneys for a longer period of time thereby increasing the radiation exposure to the kidney.

8.021 Diuretics (such as furosemide) should be administered:
   A. at the beginning of a renal study
   B. when the bladder begins to fill
   C. before the tracer leaves the kidneys
   D. after the patient voids
   E. none of the above

B. is correct.
When the bladder begins to fill, a working drainage system is demonstrated and a diuretic may be safely administered.

8.022 In evaluating acute renal failure (end-stage vs recoverable), which is the radiopharmaceutical of choice for delayed images (30 min., 4 hours, and 24 hours)?
   A. ^{99m}Tc DMSA
   B. ^{99m}Tc DTPA
   C. ^{99m}Tc GH
   D. 131 I hippuran
   E. A or D

D. is correct.
131 I hippuran is concentrated in the renal tubules and has a long half-life (T1/2P = 8.1 days) permitting 24 hour delay imaging.

8.023 Which part of the anatomy is least helpful in positioning a patient prior to injection of a radiopharmaceutical for a renal scan?
   A. xiphoid process
   B. iliac crests
   C. umbilicus
   D. costal-chondral margins

D. is correct.
The kidneys are generally located posteriorly between the umbilicus and xiphoid process as well as between the iliac crests on the sides.

8.024 Positioning the scintillation camera for a renal transplant should be:
   A. over the right or left flank
   B. anteriorly - directly under the umbilicus
   C. posteriorly - near the native kidney
   D. none of the above

D. is correct.
Renal transplants are generally positioned in the right iliac fossa; however checking the patient's history, chart, and interviewing or palpating the patient will provide the most accurate information as to location of the transplanted kidney.

8.025 Which kidney lies in the superior position?
   A. left kidney
   B. right kidney
   C. neither

A. is correct.
The right kidney lies slightly inferior to the left kidney because of displacement by the liver on the right.

8.026 The aorta is located closest to which kidney within the abdomen?
   A. nearly exactly between the kidneys
   B. right kidney
   C. left kidney

C. is correct.
The aorta can be seen on the renal flow scan next to the left kidney. The inferior vena cava is closer to the right kidney.

8.027 A normal renogram can be described as:
   A. a slow accumulation of tracer for the first 10 - 15 minutes followed by an exponential drop for 15 - 20 minutes
   B. a sharp rise in activity in the kidneys for the first few minutes followed by an exponential drop in activity for the next 20 minutes
   C. a sharp rise in renal activity in the first few minutes followed by a leveling in activity for the next 20 minutes
   D. a sharp rise in renal activity in the first few minutes followed by a slow drop in activity for the next 60 minutes

B. is correct.
Normal renograms also show equal perfusion and washout in both kidneys.

8.028 The appearance of renal artery stenosis (RAS) on a renal scan is best described as:
   A. a slow accumulation of the tracer for the first 10 -15 minutes followed by an exponential drop for 15 - 20 minutes
   B. a sharp rise in activity in the kidneys for the first few minutes followed by an exponential drop in activity for the next 20 minutes
   C. a sharp rise in renal activity in the first few minutes followed by a leveling in activity for the next 20 minutes
   D. a sharp rise in renal activity in the first few minutes followed by a slow drop in activity for the next 60 minutes

A. is correct.
RAS is an arterial blockage that prevents normal perfusion.

8.029 After the administration of furosemide, a normal renogram would show:
   A. no change in counts in the renal ROI's
   B. rapid wash-out of the kidneys
   C. rapid increase in renal counts
   D. none of the above

B. is correct.
A rapid decrease in counts in the renal ROI's would demonstrate the absence of obstruction in the renal system.

8.030 The appearance of a renal cyst on a radionuclide scan would most likely be:
   A. more perfused than the surrounding kidney
   B. photopenic, compared to surrounding kidney
   C. about the same activity as the surrounding kidney
   D. varies greatly depending on patient weight

B. is correct.
Renal cysts are usually relatively avascular and would most often have less activity than the surrounding kidney.

8.031 The procedure of the estimation of the glomerular filtration rate (GFR) includes:
   A. pre and post ^{99m}Tc DTPA injection syringe count
   B. pre and post 131 I hippuran injection syringe count
   C. injection of 131I hippuran and blood samples withdrawn for activity determination and calculations
   D. injection of ^{99m}Tc DTPA and blood samples withdrawn for activity determination and calculations
   E. none of the above

A. is correct.
The counts determined are then applied to a formula for GFR estimation.

8.032 The procedure for the estimation of effective renal plasma flow (ERPF) includes:
   A. pre and post ^{99m}Tc DTPA injection syringe count
   B. pre and post 131 I hippuran injection syringe count
   C. injection of 131I hippuran and blood samples withdrawn for activity determination and calculations
   D. injection of ^{99m}Tc DTPA and blood samples withdrawn for activity determination and calculations
   E. none of the above

C. is correct.
ERPF is estimated from blood plasma counts at specific times.

8.033 Assuming the patient has been injected properly, a correctly placed ROI on the aorta during processing would show _____ on a renal flow curve (counts vs time).
   A. rapid spike and quick exponential drop toward background after the renal activity begins
   B. rapid spike and quick exponential drop toward background before the renal activity begins
   C. gradual accumulation of the tracer just as the kidney activity appears
   D. none of the above

B. is correct.
A good bolus injection is evident when a sharp spike is noticed on the curves before the activity in the kidneys.

8.034 Two radiopharmaceuticals that can be used to measure the effective renal plasma flow (ERPF) include 131I hippuran (OIH) and:
   A. ^{99m}Tc DTPA
   B. ^{99m}Tc GH
   C. ^{99m}Tc MAG3
   D. none of the above

C. is correct.
131I hippuran and ^{99m}Tc MAG3 are removed from the bloodstream by the renal tubules. 123I hippuran is also available for ERPF determination.

8.035 Which of the following is not necessary for an ERPF (effective renal plasma flow) calculation?
   A. pre and post injection syringe counts
   B. patient's height
   C. patient's weight
   D. renal ROI counts
   E. all are needed

E. is correct.
All are necessary for the formula, including the patient's height and weight to estimate renal size.

8.036 The agent that best demonstrates the appearance of renal scarring is:
  A. ^{99m}Tc DTPA
  B. ^{99m}Tc GH
  C. ^{99m}Tc MAG3
  D. none of the above
  E. B and C

E. is correct.
^{99m}Tc GH and ^{99m}Tc MAG3 are cortical fixation agents that are best used to demonstrate scarring.

8.037 Patient preparation for renal scanning includes:
  A. NPO after midnight
  B. well - hydrated
  C. NPO 4 hours prior to injection
  D. no preparation is necessary

B. is correct.
In most cases, patients are encouraged to drink several glasses of water prior to scanning, especially with studies involving a diuretic.

8.038 Captopril renal scans are considered positive if:
  A. the post-captopril scan is unchanged from the pre-captopril scan (baseline)
  B. the post-captopril scan shows increased perfusion compared to the baseline
  C. the post-captopril scan shows decreased perfusion compared to the baseline
  D. none of the above

C. is correct.
A positive captopril scan can be said to make "a bad kidney look worse".

8.039 Nuclear cystography is imaging performed to diagnose:
  A. hydronephrosis
  B. non-functioning kidneys
  C. RAS (renal artery stenosis)
  D. ureteral reflux

D. is correct.
Nuclear cystography is used to demonstrate reflux in patients with a history of UTI's. Imaging is done pre-void, while voiding, and post-void by either ^{99m}Tc DTPA injection (indirect cystogram) or by filling the bladder directly with ^{99m}TcO4- via direct bladder catheterization.

8.040 The kidney ROI for a renogram must include the renal:
  A. calyces
  B. cortex
  C. pelvis
  D. A and B
  E. A and C
  F. B and C
  G. A, B, and C

B. is correct.
The glomeruli are located in the renal cortex and the activity determined there is necessary to calculate GFR (Glomerular Filtration Rate) and generate the renogram curves.

8.041 Radionuclide scans of renal transplants are useful in identifying:
  A. acute tubular necrosis
  B. infarction
  C. rejection
  D. all of the above
  E. none of the above

D. is correct.
Renal scans are useful as a follow-up after transplantation to evaluate the organ's function and perfusion.

8.042 Which of the following radiopharmaceuticals may also be used to differentiate renal rejection from acute renal failure?
  A. ^{99m}Tc MDP
  B. ^{99m}Tc sulfur colloid
  C. 75Se methioninie
  D. ^{99m}Tc GHA

B. is correct.
^{99m}Tc sulfur colloid has been used to detect rejection based on the fact that the inflammatory response in rejection may result in endothelial damage and local thrombosis. Uptake has been observed significantly more often in rejecting grafts than in acute tubular necrosis.

8.043 Common blood tests that are pertinent to renal function include:
   A. blood urea nitrogen (BUN)
   B. creatinine
   C. total bilirubin
   D. A and B
   E. A and C
   F. B and C
   G. A, B, and C

D. is correct.
BUN and creatinine are both waste products cleared by functioning kidneys.

8.044 On radionuclide imaging, testicular torsion is often demonstrated by:
   A. decreased flow; photopenic area on delayed imaging
   B. increased flow; photopenic area on delayed imaging
   C. increased flow; hyperperfused area on delayed images
   D. decreased flow; hyperperfused area on delayed images

A. is correct.
A later appearance of testicular torsion is the "donut sign" or hyperemia around a photopenic area.

8.045 On radionuclide imaging, epididymitis is often demonstrated by:
   A. decreased flow; photopenic area on delayed imaging
   B. increased flow; photopenic area on delayed imaging
   C. increased flow; hyperperfused area on delayed images
   D. decreased flow; hyperperfused area on delayed images

C. is correct.
Epididymitis often show hyperemia on both the flow and delayed images.

8.046 Testicular torsion is often accompanied by:
   A. blood in the urine
   B. lack of acute pain with swelling
   C. fever
   D. pain, nausea

D. is correct.
Scrotal pain, nausea, as well as swelling occurs with torsion.

8.047 Which of the following statements is true as regards the epididymis?
   A. surround both testicles, like a sac
   B. lies outside the testis, but within the scrotal sac
   C. symptoms of inflammation (epididymitis) mimic torsion
   D. A and C
   E. B and C

E. is correct.
Epididymitis presents with fever, pain, and swelling of the epididymis which is in the scrotum posterior to the testis.

8.048 In some nuclear medicine departments, _____ may be given to reduce the dose to the thyroid from ^{99m}Tc pertechnatate injected for testicular imaging.
   A. potassium permanganate
   B. potassium perchlorate
   C. potassium sulfide
   D. none of the above

B. is correct.
Potassium perchlorate (KClO4-) competitively displaces pertechnatate in the thyroid. By doing so, the amount of activity in the testes is increased.

8.049 The dose of ^{99m}Tc pertechnatate used for scrotal imaging is typically:
   A. 500 uCi
   B. 1 -2 mCi
   C. 10 - 15 mCi
   D. 20 mCi
   E. none of the above

C. is correct.
^{99m}Tc pertechnatate doses are reduced for pediatric imaging.

8.050 Which of the following protocols would maximize the counts coming from the testicles?
   A. place a lead shield over the thighs, prop testes on a towel over the shield, position camera anteriorly, inject bolus $^{99m}TcO4-$, image
   B. tape penis up on abdomen, place a lead shield over the thighs, prop testes on a towel over the shield, position camera anteriorly, inject bolus $^{99m}TcO4-$, image
   C. tape penis up on abdomen, prop testes on a towel over the shield, position camera anteriorly, inject bolus $^{99m}TcO4-$, image
   D. position camera under the testes, inject bolus $^{99m}TcO4-$, image

B. is correct.
This procedure isolates the testes and puts them in the best position for diagnostic information

8.051 Patient preparation for testicular imaging includes:
   A. hydrate patient (3 - 4 glasses water)
   B. NPO 4 hours
   C. catheter place in patient
   D. none of the above

D. is correct.
The study is done without preparation other than the patient positioning.

SECTION 9: RESPIRATORY SCINTIGRAPHY

TUTORIAL

The lungs are organs in the respiratory system that assist in the exchange of gases between the atmosphere and the blood. The overall exchange of gases between the atmosphere, blood and cells is called respiration and involves three basic processes; ventilation, or the inspiration and expiration of air between the atmosphere and the lungs, the exchange of gases between the lungs and the blood, and the exchange of gases between the blood and the cells. Respiration involves the proper functioning of both the respiratory organs and the cardiovascular system.

The lungs are cone shaped and extend from just above the clavicles (apices of the lungs) to the diaphragm (bases of the lungs). Bronchi and pulmonary vessels enter each lung at the hilum. The right lung is divided into three lobes, the left into two lobes. The ribs offer support for the intercostal muscles which along with the diaphragm are the main respiratory muscles

The gas exchange units of the lungs are the alveoli which are packed together in a "honeycomb" arrangement. Each alveolus has approximately 1000 capillaries associated with it and it is here where the exchange of respiratory gases occur. Because of the cardiovascular-respiratory function of the lungs, imaging involves two parts - the ventilation of the lungs, or evaluation of air flow, and the perfusion of the lungs, to evaluate the pulmonary arterial blood flow.

The most important clinical indication for lung ventilation/perfusion imaging is in the diagnosis of pulmonary embolism (PE) which is indicated by a compromise in the arterial blood flow to the lungs. Emboli can be the result of thrombi (usually in the deep veins of the lower extremities, especially above the knee) that break loose and embolize the pulmonary vasculature. In previously healthy individuals, the ventilation of the lungs is usually well maintained, with patent bronchial tubes. Therefore, a mismatch of defects, abnormal perfusion with normal ventilation, suggests a high probability of pulmonary embolism.

Indications for lung perfusion and ventilation studies other than PE include: chronic obstructive pulmonary disease (COPD), asthma, localized airway obstruction, bacterial, viral, or fungal infections, left heart failure, lung tumors, and metastatic lung tumors.

Radiopharmaceuticals currently in use to assess ventilation function include:

1 33Xe (xenon)gas	10-20 mCi (370-640 Mbq)	T1/2=5.3days	E=80 keV
	inhaled (gas must be trapped/filtered)	All phases of ventilation can be assessed	
81mKr (krypton) gas	1-10 mCi (37-370MBq)	T1/2=13 seconds	E=190 keV
	inhaled (81mKr gas generator -parent 81Rb is needed) Multiple projections may be		
	obtained - no equilibrium or wash-out		
99mTcDTPA aerosol	35mCi in nebulizer (<10-15% delivered to patient)		
		T1/2=6 hours	E=140 keV
	inhaled (nebulizer is need to generate aerosol) Multiple projections may be obtained -		
	no equilibrium or wash-out		

Perfusion to the lungs is assayed using 2 - 5 mCi (74 -185 MBq) of ^{99m}Tc- labeled macroaggregated albumin. Attention must be paid to patient history and manufacturers recommendations for labeling and administering. Dose and number of particles is adjusted for pediatric patients and patients with right-to-left cardiac shunts.

9.001 Which of the following statements about the lungs is(are) true?
- A. the lungs extend from slightly above the clavicles to the diaphragm
- B. the lungs function in air distribution and gas exchange
- C. the inferior surface of the lungs is called the base
- D. the lungs are cone-shaped
- E. the left lung is divided into three lobes and the right lobe into two lobes
- F. all of the above
- G. A, B, C, and D

G. is correct.
The lungs lie in the thoracic cavity, protected by the ribs, extending from just above the clavicles to the diaphragm. The broad inferior portion of the cone-shaped lungs is called the base, while the narrower superior portion is the apex. The principal function of respiration is to supply cells of the body with oxygen and remove the carbon dioxide produced by cellular activities.

9.002 The primary respiratory muscles are the:
- A. abdominal muscles and diaphragm
- B. intercostal muscles and abdominal muscles
- C. pectoralis major and diaphragm
- D. intercostal muscles and diaphragm

D. is correct.
Contraction of the principal respiratory muscles, the intercostals (external) and the diaphragm, increases lung volume and thus decreases the pressure in the lungs allowing inspiration to occur.

9.003 The site of gas exchange in the lungs is:
- A. trachea
- B. terminal bronchioles
- C. alveolar ducts
- D. alveoli

D. is correct.
The exchange of respiratory gases between the lungs and the blood takes place by diffusion across alveolar and capillary walls. The alveoli and alveolar sacs surround the alveolar ducts.

9.004 The volume of air exhaled normally after a normal inspiration is called:
- A. residual volume
- B. tidal volume
- C. total lung capacity
- D. expiratory reserve volume
- E. vital capacity

B. is correct.
Tidal volume is defined as the air that is inhaled or exhaled during normal breathing.

9.005 The largest volume of air that a person can move in and out of their lungs is called:
- A. residual volume
- B. tidal volume
- C. total lung capacity
- D. expiratory reserve volume
- E. vital capacity

E. is correct.
Vital capacity is the sum of inspiratory reserve volume, tidal volume, and expiratory reserve volume.

9.006 Which facts allow gas exchange to occur?
- A. the PO_2 of alveolar air is greater than the PO_2 of venous blood
- B. the PCO_2 of alveolar air is greater than the PCO_2 of venous blood
- C. the PCO_2 of venous blood is greater than the PCO_2 of alveolar air
- D. A and B
- E. A and C

E. is correct.
Partial pressures of the respiratory gases are important in determining the movement of oxygen and carbon dioxide between the lungs and blood and the blood and body cells. The diffusion of the gases follows the concentration gradient. In alveolar air, the PO_2 is higher than the PO_2 of venous blood; in venous blood, the PCO_2 is greater in venous blood than in alveolar air. Thus, oxygen diffuses from the alveoli to the venous blood and carbon dioxide from the venous blood to the alveoli to be exhaled.

9.007 Pulmonary blood flow in a person sitting in an upright position will be:
   A. more abundant in the base of the lungs
   B. more abundant in the apex of the lungs
   C. more abundant posteriorly than anteriorly throughout the lungs
   D. uniformly distributed throughout the lungs

A. is correct.
The upper parts of the lungs get very little blood flow while in the upright position, and increases as one approaches the bases of the lungs. In the supine position, a similar gradient exists with the posterior portions of the lungs receiving the greater amount of blood flow.

9.008 Which type of breathing pattern best describes dyspnea?
   A. normal quiet breathing
   B. labored breathing
   C. very rapid rate of breathing
   D. periodic cessation of breathing

B. is correct.
Dyspnea is an air hunger resulting in labored or difficult breathing. It may or may not be accompanied by pain.

9.009 Which blood pH would be indicative of respiratory acidosis?
   A. 7.10
   B. 7.40
   C. 7.70
   D. all of above are within normal limits

A. is correct.
Blood has a pH of 7.35 to 7.45 (7.40). As one goes lower on the pH scale, the values represented are increasingly more acidic. Blood pH of 7.10 would indicate a condition of respiratory acidosis.

9.010 The most frequent application of the lung ventilation/perfusion (V/Q) scan is:
   A. bronchogenic carcinoma
   B. pulmonary emphysema
   C. pulmonary embolis
   D. pneumonia
   E. pulmonary hypertension

C. is correct.
The diagnostic value of lung scintigraphy is best demonstrated in suspicion of pulmonary vascular occlusion, such as pulmonary embolism.

9.011 The major cause of pulmonary embolism (PE) is:
   A. trauma or injury
   B. fatty emboli from arteriosclerosis
   C. air embolism from an intravenous infusion with air in the line
   D. thrombi from deep venous thrombophlebitis
   E. pulmonary edema

D. is correct.
Thrombi that form in the deep veins of the lower extremities break loose and travel through the inferior vena cava to the right heart. Depending on their size, the emboli then may lodge in the pulmonary arterial tree or capillary bed.

9.012 Defects due to pulmonary embolism can be distinguished from those due to emphysema and carcinoma by repeat scanning. On subsequent scans, defects that are due to PE will:
   A. remain unchanged
   B. show a changing pattern
   C. become more visible
   D. none of the above

B. is correct.
Since many emboli are broken down by the body's fibrolytic system, defects due to pulmonary emboli tend to demonstrate a changing pattern over time as some of the emboli are resolved.

9.013 Because lung imaging is an effective, simple, and safe method of evaluating the state of pulmonary arterial perfusion, it can be used to:
   A. determine the presence of regional ischemia
   B. screen patients with suspected acute pulmonary embolism
   C. determine pulmonary hypertension secondary to cardiac disease
   D. all of the above

D. is correct.
Any pathology that will disrupt the arterial blood flow to the lungs may be evaluated using the non invasive lung perfusion imaging.

9.014 Which of the following statements concerning routine lung imaging is INCORRECT?

    A. Lung imaging is not as sensitive as chest radiographs in detecting pulmonary emboli

    B. Lung imaging can be altered by any condition which affects distribution of pulmonary blood flow

    C. Lung imaging cannot be interpreted without a recent chest radiograph

    D. Lung imaging is not specific for embolism

A. is correct.
Lung perfusion imaging is more sensitive than a chest radiograph which in the absence of other pathologies, would be normal in a patient with pulmonary emboli.

9.015 Negative lung perfusion images:

    A. do not exclude the possibility of major emboli

    B. excludes the possibility of major emboli

    C. excludes the possibility of any pulmonary pathology

    D. excludes the possibility of COPD

B. is correct.
Lung perfusion imaging is sensitive to any major disruption of blood flow to the lungs; absence of defects virtually excludes the possibility of pulmonary emboli.

9.016 In the absence of a ventilation scan, a segmental or lobar perfusion defect seen on ^{99m}Tc MAA perfusion scintigraphy would be _____ in the diagnosis of pulmonary embolism.

    A. both sensitive and specific

    B. sensitive, but not specific

    C. not sensitive, but specific

    D. not sensitive and non specific

    E. uninterpretable

B. is correct.
Without the ventilation scan and a recent chest x-ray, the lung perfusion scan is sensitive in demonstrating defects, but relatively non specific or equivocal in diagnosing PE.

Use the following data to answer questions 9.017 - 9.019

A patient with a suspected defect between the right and left cardiac cavities is sent for a nuclear medicine lung perfusion study. After injection, a scan of the patient's lungs, brain, and kidneys is performed. Quantitative analysis provides the following information:

Right Lung	220,000 counts	Brain	45,000 counts
Left Lung	195,000 counts	Kidneys	35,000 counts

9.017 What percentage of the radiopharmaceutical was trapped by the lungs?

    A. 44 %

    B. 53 %

    C. 84 %

    D. 89 %

C. is correct.
Total lung counts (415,000) divided by the total number of counts from all sources (495,000) times 100 = 84%.

9.018 What percent of the total activity was shunted to the systemic circulation?

    A. 7 %

    B. 10 %

    C. 16 %

    D. 19 %

C. is correct.
Total counts for brain and kidneys (80,000) divided by the total from all sources (495,000) times 100 = 16 %.

9.019 In preparing the radiopharmaceutical for this patient (right-to-left cardiac shunt) or a pediatric patient, what might the technologist need to do?

    A. increase the time from injection to imaging

    B. reduce the number of MAA particles injected

    C. increase the number of MAA particles injected

    D. inject the patient in an upright position

    E. none of the above

B. is correct.
It is optimal to reduce the number of MAA particles given because of the possibility of the MAA particles bypassing the lungs and localizing in the cerebral or renal capillaries. In pediatric patients, there are fewer capillaries and arterioles and fewer particles should be injected to reduce the risk of compromising the patient.

9.020 The radionuclide image (V/Q) of the lung, provides a map of lung:
  A. perfusion
  B. ventilation
  C. resorption
  D. all of the above
  E. A and B only

E. is correct.
When both ventilation and perfusion images are obtained, air flow (ventilation) and blood flow (perfusion) to the lungs is being assessed.

9.021 Which of the following radiopharmaceuticals has NOT been used to evaluate lung ventilation?
  A. 127 Xe
  B. 133 Xe
  C. 67 Ga
  D. 81mKr
  E. ^{99m}Tc DTPA

C. is correct.
All except 67 Ga have been used to assess lung ventilation. Xenon 127 and 133, and krypton 81m as gases, and ^{99m}Tc DTPA as an aerosol.

9.022 Perfusion lung imaging produces effective images because of:
  A. entrapment of gamma emitting radionuclide in pulmonary circulation
  B. presence of metabolically-active lesions
  C. decreased rate of pulmonary blood flow
  D. normal phagocytic function

A. is correct.
The particle size of MAA (10-90 microns) is greater than that of the capillaries in the pulmonary beds (7-10 microns) and are therefore trapped.

9.023 Sources of error in pulmonary imaging may include:
  A. patient motion
  B. normal respiration during scanning
  C. uneven perfusion due to patient's position
  D. all of the above
  E. A and C only

E. is correct.
A and C may introduce artifacts to the images that could result in erroneous reading of the scan results. Normal respiration should not produce artifacts that would affect the results of pulmonary imaging.

9.024 The mechanism for localization of pulmonary perfusion is based on:
  A. capillary blockade (clearance of radioactive particles in the capillary vasculature)
  B. the rate of disappearance of radioactive particles from systemic circulation
  C. the rate of renal excretion of radioactive particles
  D. phagocytosis of the particles by the lungs
  E. none of the above

A. is correct.
Injection of particles that are larger in size than the diameter of the capillaries will result in the particles being trapped or blocked by the capillaries in the pulmonary vasculature.

9.025 One source of error with lung imaging may be due to:
  A. pulmonary embolus
  B. drawing back on the syringe plunger before injection
  C. particles not shaken immediately before injection
  D. hypertension
  E. B and C

E. is correct.
Drawing back on the syringe allowing the patient's blood to mix with the dose and not shaking the dose before injection may cause clumping of the radiopharmaceutical and result in "hot" spots on the scan images.

9.026 What needs to be considered when injecting a dose of ^{99m}Tc MAA through plastic tubing or syringes?
  A. the proportion of dose that never reaches the patient
  B. mixing of the dose with patient blood
  C. speed of injection
  D. position of the patient
  E. all of the above

E. is correct.
Eliminating drawing back on the syringe, or allowing patient blood to mix with the dose, will prevent "clumping of the radiopharmaceutical. Using an infusion set with a saline flush will help clear the dose from the tubing, and allow a slow injection of the dose. Since gravity plays an important role in the distribution of particles, a patient in the upright position will have a greater concentration of particles at the bases of the lungs.

9.027 Lung imaging may be indicated in patients with:
  A. emphysema
  B. pulmonary hypertension
  C. carcinoma of the lung
  D. unexplained dyspnea or chest pain
  E. all of the above
  F. A and C only
  G. none of the above

E. is correct.
All are indications for lung imaging; the most common indication being pulmonary embolism.

9.028 In a normal patient lying flat, the pulmonary blood flow is:
  A. more abundant in the base of the lung
  B. more abundant in the apex of the lung
  C. uniformly distributed throughout the lung, greater toward the posterior
  D. the patient's position does not influence the pulmonary blood distribution

C. is correct.
Posture and the direction of gravity have been shown to affect the distribution of blood flow to the lungs in the normal patient.

9.029 133 Xe allows for the assessment of which of the following phase(s) of ventilation?
  A. single breath
  B. wash-in or equilibrium
  C. wash-out
  D. all of the above
  E. B and C only

D. is correct.
The use of 133Xe allows for evaluation of all phases of ventilation, single breath, equilibrium, and wash-out.

9.030 Sequential acquisitions taken while the patient exhales 133 Xe comprises the _____ portion of the test.
  A. wash-out
  B. wash-in
  C. perfusion
  D. equilibrium

A. is correct.
The wash-out phase images demonstrate clearance of the radiopharmaceutical activity from the lungs (usually within a few minutes).

9.031 Of the following, the preferred position for lung perfusion injection and imaging is:
  A. supine
  B. prone
  C. trendelenburg
  D. fetal

A. is correct.
Injecting in the supine position insures a more uniform distribution of the radiopharmaceutical. It should be noted for the reading physician what position the patient was in for injection and scanning.

9.032 Patient preparation for ^{99m}Tc microsphere lung imaging includes:
   A. an overnight fast
   B. vigorous exercise
   C. premedication with pure oxygen
   D. preparation is not required

D. is correct.
V/Q imaging can be performed on an emergency basis with no patient preparation.

9.033 Multiple views of the lungs are needed because:
   A. most collimators have a limited depth of focus
   B. each lung must be scanned separately
   C. the lungs must be scanned with the patient in sitting and supine position
   D. of the nature of particle distribution within the lung

A. is correct.
Because of the size of the lung field, multiple views of the lungs are needed to assess the entire lung field. If limited views are necessitated, the posterior and anterior views will provide the images of the largest amount of lung field. Generally, anterior, posterior, LPO, RPO, and right and left lateral views are obtained.

9.034 In pulmonary ventilation imaging:
   A. 133 Xe is inhaled
   B. 133Xe is injected
   C. ^{99m}Tc DTPA is injected
   D. 131 I is inhaled

A. is correct.
133 Xe is a radioactive gas that is inhaled to assess all phases of ventilation. ^{99m}Tc DTPA aerosol may also be inhaled for evaluation of ventilation.

9.035 Prolonged retention of 133 Xe in regions of the lung correspond to:
   A. obstructive lung disease
   B. reduced trapping of particles in the lungs
   C. pulmonary emboli
   D. pneumonia
   E. right-to-left shunt

A. is correct.
Obstructive lung disease is demonstrated on the 133Xe wash-out images as prolonged or delayed clearance.

9.036 If 133 Xe ventilation imaging is performed after ^{99m}Tc MAA imaging, which of the following will degrade the quality of the images?
   A. off peak window needed for perfusion study
   B. decreased dose for the perfusion study
   C. upscatter of 133 Xe
   D. downscatter of ^{99m}Tc

D. is correct.
Downscatter of the higher energy (140 keV) photons into the lower energy (80 keV) xenon will degrade the image.

9.037 Drawbacks to 133Xe ventilation imaging include all of the following EXCEPT:
   A. low gamma photon energy (80 keV)
   B. a trap or exhaust is needed to remove the gas
   C. all phases of ventilation can be assessed
   D. patient cooperation is essential

C. is correct.
Assessment of all phases of ventilation is an advantage that is not shared by other radiopharmaceuticals currently in use for ventilation studies. The low gamma energy results in an increase in soft tissue attenuation and thereby decreased resolution. If 133 Xe imaging is performed after the perfusion study using ^{99m}Tc MAA, downscatter from the ^{99m}Tc into the 133 Xe window degrades the image quality.

9.038 All of the following are advantages of 81mKr lung ventilation imaging EXCEPT:
- A. ventilation studies can be performed after the perfusion study
- B. 81mKr images may be taken in multiple projections
- C. 81m Kr may be used on portable studies in the intensive care unit
- D. there is no need to trap or exhaust the gas
- E. single breath and wash-out images are not possible

E. is correct.
Because of its energy (190 keV) and half-life (13 seconds), 81mKr has several advantages. The 190 keV energy makes it possible to perform the ventilation study after the perfusion study. When looking for PE, a negative perfusion study would preclude the necessity for ventilation imaging. There is no need to trap the krypton because of its extremely short half-life, so portable studies can be done on patients on respirators. When perfusion defects are demonstrated, the ventilation study using 81mKr can be accomplished in the views that best demonstrated the defect on perfusion imaging.

9.039 ^{99m}Tc DTPA aerosol is deposited in the bronchial tree in relation to:
- A. air flow rate
- B. particle size
- C. turbulence
- D. all of above

D. is correct.
Because of its dependence on air flow rates, particle size, and turbulence of flow, the aerosol study requires attention to all variables affecting the procedure.

9.040 Multiple projections of the lungs may be obtained with ^{99m}Tc DTPA aerosol.
- A. true
- B. false

A. is correct.
An advantage over conventional 133 Xe gas ventilation studies, ^{99m}Tc DTPA aerosol allows multiple images to be obtained in the same projections as the perfusion images.

9.041 The nuclear medicine technologist notices the appearance of esophagus and stomach on a DTPA aerosol ventilation scan. The most appropriate response is to:
- A. prepare a new kit of DTPA and re-administer to the patient
- B. check the particle size of the aerosol
- C. continue the scan; this is a typical finding
- D. change the tubing and check the nebulizer for cracks
- E. have the patient hold their breath during re-administration of the dose

C. is correct.
The appearance of stomach and esophagus results from the patient swallowing the DTPA aerosol during the inhalation. This is a typical finding.

9.042 Patients with obstructive pulmonary disease may show an aerosol scan appearance:
- A. that mimics the appearance of pulmonary emboli
- B. that results in central airway deposition of the radiopharmaceutical
- C. that results in a false negative study
- D. all of the above

B. is correct.
Obstructive pulmonary disease may prevent the aerosol particles from penetrating to the ends of the lung field, resulting in deposition of the DTPA particles in the central airways seen as multiple "hot" spots in the lung fields.

9.043 81mKr, 133Xe, 127Xe, and ^{99m}TcDTPA are all administered via inhalation.
- A. true
- B. false

A. is correct.
81mKr, 133Xe, and 127Xe (expensive, not readily available) are all gases and are inhaled by the patient. They require patient education and cooperation for a successful study. ^{99m}TcDTPA is an aerosol that is inhaled by the patient during normal tidal breathing.

9.044 Interpretation of V/Q scans requires that:
   A. a recent (less than 4 hours) chest radiograph be evaluated
   B. the patient not be in respiratory distress
   C. a pulmonary arteriogram be scheduled
   D. the technologist and interpreting physician have knowledge of the patient's clinical status
   E. all of the above
   F. A and D

F. is correct.
A recent chest x-ray is necessary for the proper interpretation of the lung scan. The patient's clinical history is important in the evaluation of any diagnostic imaging test and will assist both the technologist and the physician in achieving the highest quality results from the nuclear medicine V/Q scan.

9.045 Interpretation of the chest radiograph, ventilation scan, and perfusion images for a typical finding of pulmonary embolism would most likely be found in:
   A. non-segmental perfusion defects, normal ventilation, abnormal chest x-ray
   B. segmental perfusion defects, normal ventilation, normal chest x-ray
   C. normal perfusion, segmental ventilation defects, normal chest x-ray
   D. normal to complete absence of perfusion in an entire lobe, patchy ventilation defects, abnormal chest x-ray

B. is correct.
This is a "classic" scan pattern for pulmonary embolis (PE). A mismatch between the perfusion and ventilation study and chest film (perfusion defects, normal ventilation and chest film) places the patient at "high probability" for pulmonary embolism.

SECTION 10: THYROID SCINTIGRAPHY

TUTORIAL

The thyroid gland consists of two lobes connected by an isthmus and is located at the base of the neck between the lower part of the larynx and the upper part of the trachea. Sometimes a third lobe, or pyramidal lobe extends upward from the isthmus. The thyroid hormones, T4 (thyroxine) and T3 (triiodothyronine) are manufactured by the follicular cells of the thyroid. While thyroxine is secreted in greater quantity, triiodothyronine is 3 to 4 times more metabolically potent. The thyroid hormones have three principal effects on the body: Regulation of metabolism; regulation of growth and development, and regulation of the activity of the nervous system.

Hyposecretion of thyroxine leads to a condition of mental and physical sluggishness, which is called myxedema in the adult. Hyposecretion during the growth years results in cretinism. Hyperthyroidism is the state in which tissues are responding to an oversecretion of thyroid hormone.

Thyroid hormone production is controlled by a negative feedback system involving the hypothalamus, pituitary and thyroid glands. Thyroid stimulating hormone, or TSH, (secreted by the anterior pituitary gland) stimulates release of thyroid hormones from the thyroid gland. Increased circulating hormone will signal a suppression of TSH, while a decrease will cause more TSH to stimulate the thyroid to produce and secrete more thyroid hormone. The hypothalamus secretes thyrotropin releasing factor (TRF) which stimulates the anterior pituitary to secrete TSH. Measurement of TSH is an indicator of the effect of the thyroid hormone on the body's tissues.

Tests in nuclear medicine take advantage of the localization mechanism of iodine as it is trapped by the thyroid gland. For routine imaging procedures, 123I or ^{99m}Tc pertechnate are used. In vivo tests of thyroid function (e.g. thyroid uptake) use 131I, 123I, or ^{99m}Tc pertechnatate. While the 131I and 123I are usually ingested (as a capsule), ^{99m}Tc pertechnatate is injected intravenously. Normal ranges for thyroid uptake should be established in each department for the radionuclide of choice.

Indications for thyroid imaging include the evaluation of relative functions of palpable nodules and the location of thyroid tissue in locations outside the thyroid bed. Metastases of thyroid cancer may be present nearly anywhere in the body.

A thorough patient history should be obtained for symptoms, previous surgeries, and medications or procedures that could affect the uptake and image results. The uptake is performed with a flat field collimator if 131I or 123I is used and a parallel hole collimator if ^{99m}Tc pertechnatate is used. Imaging is usually accomplished in the anterior, and right and left anterior obliques.

10.001 The lobes of the thyroid are connected by the:
   A. thyroid cartilage
   B. thyroglossal duct
   C. isthmus
   D. pyramidal lobe

C. is correct.
The isthmus is thyroid tissue connecting the right and left lateral lobes of the thyroid, lying anterior to the trachea, below the cricoid cartilage.

10.002 The lobes of the thyroid are usually of _____ size and _____ lobe is larger.
   A. unequal; left
   B. equal; neither
   C. equal; right
   D. unequal; right

D. is correct.
The right lobe is often slightly larger than the left lobe.

10.003 TRF (thyrotropin releasing factor) is secreted in the:
   A. thyroid
   B. hypothalamus
   C. hypophyseal portal system
   D. anterior pituitary

B. is correct.
Secreted by the hypothalamus, TRF is a hormone that stimulates the anterior pituitary to produce TSH.

10.004 The anterior pituitary produces:
   A. thyroxine (T4)
   B. monoiodotyrosine (MIT)
   C. TSH
   D. TRF

C. is correct.
TSH (thyroid stimulating hormone) is also called thyrotropin and is secreted by the anterior pituitary gland.

10.005 Steps in thyroid hormone production start with trapping (concentrating) of iodide in the thyroid follicular cells followed by:
   A. organification; release
   B. trapping; organification
   C. organification; washout
   D. organification; coupling

D. is correct.
After trapping or concentration of the iodide, the iodide is organified (oxidized) to form MIT or DIT. Coupling of one MIT molecule and one DIT molecule forms T3, while the coupling of two DIT molecules forms T4. These hormones are stored in the gland until signaled for release by TSH.

10.006 Iodine trapping can be competitively blocked by the administration of:
   A. pertechnetate ($^{99m}TcO4-$)
   B. potassium perchlorate (KClO4-)
   C. A and B
   D. none of the above

C. is correct.
Both pertechnetate and perchlorate anions compete with iodine for trapping sites in the thyroid gland.

10.007 Which of the two main thyroid hormones is present in higher concentration in the blood plasma?
   A. TSH
   B. T3 (triiodothyronine)
   C. T4 (thyroxine)
   D. thyrotropin

C. is correct.
Most of the stored and secreted thyroid hormone is in the form of T4.

10.008 During organification, iodide is ____ to iodine and incorporated into _____.
   A. oxidized; thyroxine
   B. oxidized; tyrosine
   C. reduced; thyroxine
   D. reduced; T4

B. is correct.
Iodotyrosines are synthesized and coupled within large molecules of glycoprotein called thyroglobulin.

10.009 Following organification, coupling of MIT and DIT takes place resulting in the production of:
A. thyroglobulin
B. triiodothyronine
C. thyroid binding globulin
D. thyroxine
E. B and D

E. is correct.
Coupling of one MIT molecule and one DIT molecule forms T3, while the coupling of two DIT molecules forms T4.

10.010 In the bloodstream, T3 and T4 are bound to:
A. thyroglobulin
B. thyroid binding globulin
C. albumin
D. B and C

D. is correct.
T3 and T4 are bound to TBG (thyroid binding globulin) and T4 is also bound to albumin and pre-albumin.

10.011 Approximately _____ percent of the administered dose of ^{99m}Tc pertechnatate is taken up by the thyroid necessitating a _____ patient dose relative to iodine.
A. .5 to 3.75; higher
B. 5 to 7; higher
C. 12 to 14; lower
D. 10 to 15; lower

A. is correct.
Although the recommended dose for imaging is higher with ^{99m}Tc pertechnetate, the thyroid absorbed radiation dose (mrad/uCi) is considerably lower.

10.012 A nodule which appears "cold" (photopenic) on a ^{99m}Tc pertechnatate scan will appear _____ on an iodine scan.
A. hyperperfused ("hot")
B. photopenic ("cold")
C. may be either A or B

B. is correct.
All radiopharmaceuticals used for thyroid imaging localize in the gland and compete for trapping sites in the same way that iodine is trapped in the gland. A "cold" or hypofunctioning nodule will not trap the radiopharmaceuticals used in imaging.

10.013 A functioning or "hot" nodule on a pertechnatate scan will appear _____ on an iodine scan.
A. hyperperfused ("hot")
B. photopenic ("cold")
C. may be either A or B

C. is correct.
A nodule which appears "hot " or at least the same intensity as the surrounding tissue on a pertechnatate scan may owe its appearance to increased trapping of pertechnatate, which would correspond to a "hot" nodule on an iodine image. In a small number of cases, however, the increased activity is due to hypervascular non-functioning tissue which would appear as a photopenic area on the iodine scan.

10.014 The recommended dose of ^{99m}Tc pertechnatate for thyroid imaging is:
A. 500 - 1500 uCi
B. 1 - 3 mCi
C. 5 - 10 mCi
D. 15 - 20 mCi

C. is correct.
The recommended dose for thyroid imaging with pertechnatate is 5 - 10 mCi (185 - 370 MBq).

10.015 Patients with chronic thyroiditis who have not been on drugs which block hormone synthesis may show a _____ uptake with pertechnatate than with iodine.
A. lower
B. higher

B. is correct.
In chronic thyroiditis, increased trapping takes place without organification. Pertechnatate, while not organified, is trapped more aggressively than iodine. In the absence of drugs which block hormone synthesis (e.g. PTU, propylthiouricil; Tapazole, Methimazole) , this is diagnostic of thyroiditis.

10.016 To determine if thyroid function is under physiologic control or autonomous activity, a _____ test would be performed.
  A. Thyroid uptake
  B. TSH stimulation
  C. T3 suppression
  D. perchlorate washout

C. is correct.
In the presence of a normal response of the thyroid gland to suppression, hyperthyroidism can be ruled out.

10.017 Which of the following may result in a decreased thyroid uptake value?
  A. Grave's disease
  B. Autoimmune thyroiditis
  C. Toxic nodular goiter
  D. TSH secretion
  E. A and C

B. is correct.
Autoimmune thyroiditis or Hashimoto's disease is the most common cause of hypothyroidism .

10.018 The condition known as myxedema results from:
  A. hyperthyroidism
  B. hypothyroidism

B. is correct.
Myxedema results from the hypofunction of the thyroid gland and is characterized by a dry, waxy swelling with distinctive facial changes.

10.019 A patient is given a 131I NaI capsule of 10 uCi. Uptake values are obtained at 2,6, and 24 hours. A 10uCi capsule is counted as a control. The interval net counts are

Time (hours)	Patient (CPM)	Control (CPM)
2	10,258	54,296
6	25,963	52,871
24	7,731	49,592

This data indicates that the patient is:
  A. hypothyroid
  B. euthyroid
  C. hyperthyroid

C. is correct.
The uptake value at 6 hours is nearly 50% indicating a hyperactive gland. The value falls to a normal range at 24 hours which may be due to the rapid turnover of the gland due to its hyperactivity.

10.020 Which of the following sites in the body are known to concentrate pertechnetate to a level greater than that of plasma?
  A. salivary glands
  B. gastric mucosa
  C. choroid plexus
  D. thymus gland
  E. pancreas
  F. A, B, and C

F. is correct.
Pertechnetate ions in the interstitial fluids are removed by only a few organ systems, the stomach, salivary glands, thyroid, bowel, choroid plexus, and kidneys.

10.021 If a patient's thyroid gland is too large to be adequately shielded for a blood background for a thyroid uptake test,:
  A. the room background can be substituted
  B. the background can be obtained over the thigh
  C. a pre-dose background may be substituted
  D. a background may be taken over the heart
  E. the background should still be taken over the neck to maintain counting geometry

B. is correct.
If a lead thyroid shield is not used, the probe is positioned vertically over the thigh, above the patient's knee, to exclude activity from the bladder.

10.022 A clinically hypothyroid patient has a low TSH level for that condition. To what can this finding be related?
   A. thyroid dysfunction
   B. hypothalamic dysfunction
   C. pituitary dysfunction
   D. B and C

D. is correct.
TSH level may become subnormal with severe disease of the pituitary or hypothalamus.

10.023 Which of the following substances will falsely decrease the RAIU (radioactive iodine uptake) value?
   A. perchlorate
   B. iodinated x-ray contrast media
   C. thyroid replacement therapy
   D. turnips and cabbage
   E. all of the above

E. is correct.
The 24 hour uptake would be increased in areas of iodine deficiency and decreased in patients with increased dietary iodine or goitrogenic foods such as turnips and cabbage, recent contrast x-rays studies, or intake of exogenous thyroid hormone.

10.024 A solitary "cold" nodule on a radioiodine scan could be:
   A. colloid cyst
   B. primary thyroid carcinoma
   C. adenoma
   D. A and B
   E. all of the above

E. is correct.
Most nodules, including those of cystic or benign nature, are hypofunctioning.

10.025 The presence of multiple "cold" areas on the thyroid scan usually indicates a _____ risk of malignancy than with a solitary lesion.
   A. significantly higher
   B. significantly lower
   C. unchanged

B. is correct.
Generally, a solitary, non-functioning ("cold") nodule is an indication for needle biopsy of the lesion and is suspicious for thyroid carcinoma.

10.026 Patients with a history of head and neck irradiation are at _____ risk for thyroid carcinoma.
   A. increased
   B. decreased
   C. unchanged

A. is correct.
Patients previously treated with radiation to the head and neck for acne, thymus enlargement, tonsils, etc., are at a higher risk for developing thyroid carcinoma. This treatment protocol was popular in the late 1940's and early 1950's with doses to the thyroid ranging from 100-300 rads.

10.027 Functioning thyroid tissue is sometimes found:
   A. at the base of the tongue
   B. along the esophagus
   C. in the mediastinum
   D. all of the above
   E. A and C only

D. is correct.

10.028 Indication(s) for thyroid scanning is(are):
   A. presence of palpable abnormality
   B. presence of ectopic thyroid tissue
   C. following thyroidectomy to determine extent and location of residual functioning thyroid tissue
   D. all of the above
   E. B and C only

D. is correct.
Radionuclide thyroid imaging is helpful for virtually all disorders of the thyroid gland whether anatomic or physiologic.

10.029 The usual route of administration of radioiodine for a thyroid uptake test is:
  A. intrathyroidal
  B. intrathecal
  C. intravenous
  D. oral

D. is correct.
Radioiodine in capsule or in solution form is administered orally for uptake purposes.

10.030 Exophthalmos is characteristic of which condition(s)?
  A. Grave's disease
  B. thyrotoxicosis
  C. hyperthyroidism
  D. all of the above
  E. A and C only

D. is correct.
Abnormal protrusion of the eye (exopthalmos) commonly occurs in A, B, and C which are synonyms of the same condition.

10.031 The presence of LATS (long acting thyroid stimulator) may be an indication of which of the following?
  A. thyroiditis
  B. Graves disease
  C. toxic nodular goiter
  D. all of the above
  E. A and B only

E. is correct.
The absence of LATS is used to differentiate toxic nodular goiter (Plummer's disease) from Graves disease and other autoimmune diseases.

10.032 The radiopharmaceutical of choice for performing a pediatric thyroid uptake is:
  A. 123 I sodium iodide
  B. 127 I sodium iodide
  C. 131 I sodium iodide
  D. ^{99m}Tc pertechnatate

A. is correct.
The radiation dose to the pediatric patient from 123 I is approximately 100 times less than from 131I.

10.033 Multinodular goiter is also known as:
  A. struma
  B. deQuervain's disease
  C. Plummer's disease
  D. Reidel's disease

C. is correct.

10.034 The etiology of Hashimoto's thyroiditis is:
  A. exogenous iodine intake
  B. viral
  C. autoimmune
  D. hypothalamic dysfunction

C. is correct.
Hashimoto's thyroiditis or autoimmune thyroiditis appear to involve antibodies that block the TSH receptors in the thyroid gland.

10.035 Graves disease is five times more prevalent in _____ than in _____.
  A. teens; adults
  B. women; men
  C. men; women

B. is correct.
In nongoitrous areas the ratio may be as high as 7:1.

10.036 Errors in measurement of the thyroid gland made when using a pinhole collimator may occur due to:
  A. long acquisition time
  B. small matrix size
  C. incorrect orientation
  D. parallax error
  E. all of the above

D. is correct.
When the distance of the gland to the pinhole is equal to that of the pinhole to the detector, a 1:1 relationship of size exists. Movement closer or further away results in over or under estimation of size.

10.037 Which of the following radiophamaceuticals can be use to image the thyroid in a patient on thyroid medication such as synthroid?
  A. 201 Tl
  B. 123 I
  C. 131 I
  D. ^{99m}Tc pertechnatate

A. is correct.
Uptake in the thyroid is less affected using a "flow" agent such as 201 Tl.

10.038 Patients being treated for thyroid disorders with exogenous T3 or synthroid should have those medications discontinued for at least _____ before obtaining a radioiodine uptake and scan.
  A. 3 - 5 days
  B. 1 week
  C. 3 weeks
  D. 1 - 2 months

C. is correct.
If greater than physiologic doses of hormone have been administered, longer periods of discontinuance may be required.

10.039 Which of the following is usually used to distinguish between a cystic and solid lesion identified as a "cold" lesion on a radionuclide thyroid scan?
  A. fine needle aspiration
  B. ultrasonography
  C. palpation
  D. open biopsy

B. is correct.
One of the strengths of sonography is its success in differentiating solid from cystic nodules both of which could be a cause of nonspecific, nonfunctioning nodules seen on thyroid scans.

10.040 A midline of activity on a ^{99m}Tc pertechnatate thyroid scan is most likely:
  A. accessory lobe
  B. sublingual extension
  C. esophageal activity
  D. ectopic salivary gland

C. is correct.
An image taken after the patient is given a sip of water will help determine if this is activity in the esophagus or pyramidal lobe of the thyroid.

10.041 Activity seen at the base of the tongue on a radioiodine thyroid scan could be:
  A. lipoma
  B. cyst
  C. fibroma
  D. sublingual thyroid
  E. all of the above

D. is correct.
Functioning thyroid tissue will take up the radioactive iodine. A mass at the base of the tongue could be a lipoma, cyst, fibroma or sublingual thyroid.

10.042 Of the following, which will suppress thyroid uptake for the longest period of time?
  A. synthroid
  B. cough medications
  C. IVP contrast
  D. oral cholecystographic agents

D. is correct.
Cholecystographic agents may take from 4 weeks to several months for excretion from the body. The others listed are excreted within 2 - 4 weeks.

10.043 Occasionally, a thyroid nodule will appear "hot" or "normal" on a ^{99m}Tc pertechnatate scan and "cold" on an iodine scan. This may be best explained by the fact that:
  A. the nodule did not organify the iodine
  B. the nodule did not trap the pertechnatate
  C. the nodule organified the iodine
  D. The nodule trapped the iodine

A. is correct.
The nodule may trap or concentrate the radionuclides, but did not organify the iodine, indicating a nonfunctioning thyroid nodule.

10.044 Congenital hypothyroidism or lack of thyroid hormone secretion results in a condition known as:
  A. Hashimoto's thyroiditis
  B. Down's syndrome
  C. Cretinism
  D. fetal distress syndrome

C. is correct.
Cretinism is the arrested physical and mental development due to congenital lack of thyroid secretion.

10.045 In the human fetus, the thyroid gland becomes functional during the:
  A. first month of gestation
  B. third month of gestation
  C. sixth month of gestation
  D. ninth month of gestation

B. is correct.
The thyroid gland is complete at three - month gestation, after which the thyroid hormones are synthesized and secreted.

10.046 Which of the following radiopharmaceuticals may be used to detect the presence of metastatic thyroid carcinoma?
  A. 201 Tl chloride
  B. 131 I
  C. ^{99m}Tc sestimibi
  D. 131 I mIBG
  E. all of the above
  F. A and B only
  G. B and C only

E. is correct.
All of the radiopharmaceuticals have been used for metastatic searches for thyroid carcinoma. Papillary and follicular carcinomas take up 131 I; 201Tl, 131 I, and ^{99m}Tc sestimibi seem to have better sensitivity for medullary carcinoma.

10.047 Patient preparation for the whole body 131I study for thyroid metastases includes all of the following EXCEPT:
  A. NPO for at least 4 hours prior to administration of dose
  B. off thyroid hormones
  C. cleansing enemas or laxatives
  D. no IV or intrathecal iodinated contrast materials for at least 3 weeks
  E. A and C only

C. is correct.
The patient should be off thyroxine (T4) for at least 4 weeks, triiodothyronine (T3) for at least 10 days. It is believed that this will increase the avidity of the thyroid metastases for the 131I. Iodinated contrast should be avoided for a least 3 weeks prior to scanning, and the patient should be NPO 4 hours prior and for a least 1 hour after administration of the 131I.

10.048 The dose of 131I for whole body scintigraphy for thyroid metastases is _____ and is administered _____.
  A. 5 -10 mCi; intravenous
  B. 5 - 10 mCi; oral
  C. 30 mCi; intravenous
  D. 30 mCi; oral

B. is correct.
The dose is in the range of 5-10 mCi (185 - 370 MBq) and is administered orally in the form of sodium iodide. Images are taken at 24-48 hours after ingestion of the radiopharmaceutical.

10.049 An advantage of 201Tl over 131I in imaging whole body metastatic thyroid is that the 201 Tl:
  A. is more sensitive than 131I
  B. has lower background of radioactivity in the abdomen
  C. does not require the patient to be off thyroid medications
  D. can be injected into the patient intravenously

C. is correct.
Concentrations of 201 Tl chloride are non-specific and imaging is usually confined to the neck and chest because of high background radioactivity. However, it can be used when the patient is still on thyroid medications because the localization mechanism is different than for 131I.

10.050 If an area of increased activity is demonstrated on a whole body 131I metastatic survey in the area of the lower pelvis or upper thigh, the technologist should:

A. consult the nuclear medicine physician for further views

B. have the patient remove clothing from that area and wash the skin

C. have the patient return for delayed views

D. have the patient drink several glasses of water

B. is correct.

Contaminations from urine can show up as localized areas of activity. The patient should wash the skin in that area and remove clothing that may be contaminated by urine. The technologist should reimage the same area after the removal of clothing and washing.

SECTION 11: LIVER AND HEPATOBILIARY SCINTIGRAPHY

TUTORIAL

The hepatobiliary system consists of the liver, gallbladder, and biliary ducts leading to the duodenum. The left and right hepatic ducts join to form the common hepatic duct which joins with the cystic duct to connect with the gallbladder. At this point the common hepatic duct becomes the common bile duct and continues to the duodenum where in approximately 70% of patients the common bile duct and main pancreatic duct enter the duodenum at the ampulla of Vater. A muscular sphincter called the sphincter of Oddi exists at the entrance to the duodenum.

Arterial blood is carried to the liver through the hepatic artery which carries oxygenated blood to the cells of the liver. The portal venous system delivers blood with nutrients from the gut to the liver and is responsible for approximately 70% of the liver perfusion.

The hepatic cells (or hepatocytes) secrete bile; the gallbladder concentrates and stores it. Kupffer cells in the liver are a part of the reticuloendothelial system (RES) and phagocytize particles that flow through the liver.

Liver scintigraphy is performed using either ^{99m}Tc sulfur colloid or ^{99m}Tc human albumin microspheres which are phagocytized by the Kupffer cells in the liver and are evenly distributed. Disease processes will affect the blood supply to the liver and will affect the distribution of the radiocolloids. Abnormalities would be visualized as a decreased area of uptake and are unspecific. Administration of ^{99m}Tc labeled RBCs will help to interpret metastatic lesions and hemangiomas because of the increased blood flow in metastases relative to normal tissue. Ultrasound and computed tomography (CT) are generally done to enhance correct diagnosis. The usual dose of radiocolloid is generally in the range of 5-12 mCi (185-444 MBq), with the higher doses used if SPECT is performed as part of the study.

Iminodiacetic acid (IDA) agents are used for hepatobiliary scintigraphy. These agents are easy to prepare, are rapidly cleared from the bloodstream by the hepatocytes by a transport mechanism that is similar to bilirubin. The primary indication for hepatobiliary imaging is to aid in the diagnosis of acute cholecystitis. Patient preparation includes having the patient NPO for at least 2 hours before the examination. A recent meal may cause the gallbladder to contract and result in a false positive study. Morphine induces contraction of the sphincter of Oddi and may enhance gallbladder visualization and shorten the procedure. Dosage of the ^{99m}Tc IDA is in the range of 5-7 mCi (185- 259 MBq). A normal study would demonstrate liver at 5 minutes with hepatic bile ducts and gallbladder visualized at 10-15 minutes with small intestine activity at 30-60 minutes. A normal study would include visualization of the gallbladder and small bowel within the hour. The absence of activity at 1 hour necessitates delayed imaging of up to 4 hours.

11.001 Decreased or absent uptake of radionuclide by portions of the liver is consistent with:
    A. metastatic disease
    B. traumatic injury
    C. impaired hepatic circulation
    D. all of the above
    E. A and B

D. is correct.
Uptake of radiocolloids by the liver is by the Kupffer cells which phagocytize particles in the blood. Space occupying lesions or injury will appear as decreased or absent uptake. As hepatocytes are destroyed by disease, hepatic circulation is dramatically altered and delivery of the colloid to the Kupffer cells is affected.

11.002 Total hepatic blood flow differs from functional or effective blood flow in that:
    A. the former includes all the blood entering the liver
    B. the latter includes all the blood which enters the liver sinusoids and allows the RES cells to function
    C. the latter refers to only the oxygenated blood entering the liver
    D. all of the above
    E. A and B only

E. is correct.
Total hepatic blood flow includes the oxygenated blood entering from the hepatic artery and the hepatic portal vein which delivers nutrients to the liver.

11.003 The liver is supplied with blood by the:
    A. portal vein
    B. mesenteric vein
    C. hepatic artery
    D. all of the above
    E. A and C only

E. is correct.
The liver has a dual blood supply. Arterial blood is delivered to the liver through the hepatic artery, the portal system carries blood from the gut to the liver and spleen.

11.004 Colloids with particles larger than one micron are not suitable for hepatic blood flow measurements because large numbers of particles are trapped in the:
    A. spleen
    B. lungs
    C. liver
    D. bone marrow
    E. kidneys

B. is correct.
If particle size is well above the 1 um size, trapping will occur in the pulmonary system through the mechanism of capillary blockade.

11.005 The liver is made up mainly of:
    A. endothelial cells
    B. polyhedral parenchymal hepatic cells
    C. kupffer cells
    D. endodermal cells

B. is correct.
The hepatocytes are responsible for a variety of liver functions including bile formation.

11.006 The parenchymal hepatic cells or hepatocytes:
    A. store glycogen, neutral fats and vitamins
    B. detoxify many substances
    C. secrete bile
    D. A and B only
    E. all of the above

E. is correct.
All of the above functions are performed by the liver hepatic cells.

11.007 Liver and spleen imaging is useful in:
    A. evaluating organ shape, size, and position
    B. detecting lesions such as malignancy and cyst
    C. evaluation of hepatitis or cirrhosis
    D. all of the above
    E. A and C only

D. is correct.
Functional liver disease can be evaluated with liver and spleen scintigraphy as well as localizing lesions and evaluating size and shape of the organs.

11.008 Kupffer cells, a part of the RES (reticuloendthelial system) play a role in:
   A. antibody formation
   B. phagocytizing foreign particles
   C. breaking down blood pigments for bile formation
   D. all of the above
   E. B and C

B. is correct.
Kupffer cells, which account for approximately 15% of the cells in the liver, have phagocytic action.

11.009 Radionuclides in colloidal forms are used for hepatic imaging because:
   A. they are phagocytized by the reticuloendothelial system
   B. they are retained by the parenchymal system
   C. they can be used to determine the patency of the bile duct
   D. they can be used to delineate gall stones
   E. all of the above
   F. both A and C

A. is correct.
The Kupffer cells remove the colloid particles from circulation. Approximately 75 - 80% of the particles are taken up by the liver, 10 - 15% by the spleen, and the rest mostly in bone marrow.

11.010 If the mean particle size of the radiocolloid prepared for liver and spleen scintigraphy is reduced:
   A. spleen uptake is reduced
   B. spleen uptake is increased
   C. bone marrow uptake is reduced
   D. bone marrow uptake is increased
   E. both A and D
   F. uptake is not affected by particle size

E. is correct.
The spleen tends to accumulate larger particles and the bone marrow, smaller particles. If the mean size is reduced, the uptake will be in the direction of the bone marrow.

11.011 Patient preparation for a ^{99m}Tc sulfur colloid imaging study includes:
   A. overnight fast
   B. a special test meal
   C. blocking of the thyroid with Lugol's solution
   D. premedication with potassium perchlorate
   E. no patient preparation is necessary

E. is correct.
No patient preparation is necessary other than insuring from patient history if any type of barium study has been performed. Barium in the colon could result in a false positive study from the attenuation and scattering of photons by the barium.

11.012 The rate of removal of a tagged colloid from hepatic circulation reflects:
   A. the state of blood flow in the liver
   B. functional efficiency of parenchymal cells
   C. the biological half - life of the radionuclide
   D. none of the above

A. is correct.
Any disease process that affects the perfusion to the liver will affect the delivery of the radiocolloid to the Kupffer cells of the liver.

11.013 Of the two main lobes of the liver:
   A. the right lobe is much larger than the left
   B. the left lobe is much larger than the right

A. is correct.
The right and left lobes are separated by the falciform ligament with the right lobe being larger than the left. The quadrate lobe and caudate lobe are associated with the right lobe of the liver.

11.014 Barium studies should not precede liver imaging since barium:
- A. falsely stimulates liver function
- B. scatters gamma photons yielding false photopenic areas
- C. will cause the tagged material to accumulate in the gall bladder
- D. will cause some portions to hyperfunction giving false "hot" areas

B. is correct.
Patients scheduled for both a liver-spleen scan and a barium study should have the nuclear medicine study performed first.

11.015 When imaging the liver for metastatic carcinoma:
- A. anterior view only is sufficient
- B. anterior and posterior views are sufficient
- C. SPECT imaging should be used routinely
- D. liver imaging is not indicated in a patient with suspected metastatic carcinoma

C. is correct.
SPECT imaging increases the accuracy of defining space occupying lesions by increasing contrast resolution and the ability to detect small lesions, both superficial and deep in the liver parenchyma.

11.016 Lacerations of the liver or spleen are usually seen as:
- A. space-occupying lesions
- B. "hot" spots
- C. convexities

A. is correct.
A defect in the spleen as from injury, may be seen as a discontinuity of the radiotracer along the border of the spleen or within the tissue itself.

11.017 Spleen imaging can demonstrate:
- A. splenic size, shape, and position
- B. decreased phagocytic activity resulting from major infections
- C. space-occupying lesions
- D. all of the above
- E. A and C only

D. is correct.
The phagocytic function of the spleen can be demonstrated with radiocolloids and tagged ^{99m}Tc RBCs that have been denatured. The spleen can be evaluated for all of the above and by diseases affecting the blood flow to the spleen.

11.018 If only three views can be obtained during spleen imaging the best views to obtain are:
- A. anterior, left and right laterals
- B. posterior, left and right laterals
- C. anterior, posterior, and right lateral
- D. anterior, posterior, and left lateral

D. is correct.
A complete spleen exam would include anterior, posterior, left lateral, and posterior oblique views to separate the liver fully from the spleen. A marker image for size would also be obtained.

11.019 Accessory spleen tissue can be found anywhere in the abdomen but is most frequently found in the:
- A. left upper quadrant
- B. left lower quadrant
- C. right upper quadrant
- D. right lower quadrant

A. is correct.
Accessory splenic tissue is most often found as splenic tissue nodules near the spleen or spleen bed if regrowth occurs after splenectomy.

11.020 Which of the following is the best view to be used in determining spleen size?
- A. anterior
- B. posterior
- C. left lateral
- D. right lateral

B. is correct.
The spleen is located in the posterior portion of the left upper abdomen and is usually more clearly seen in the posterior projection.

11.021 Regions with little or no radioactivity during spleen imaging may be due to:
   A. tumor
   B. cyst or abscess
   C. infarct
   D. all of these
   E. A and B only

D. is correct.
Any pathology that disrupts the function of the spleen will result in decreased uptake of the radiotracer by the RES system.

11.022 Which is the last organ to be visualized during liver/spleen perfusion imaging?
   A. kidneys
   B. liver
   C. heart
   D. spleen

B. is correct.
The spleen is perfused by the splenic artery off the celiac trunk of the aorta. The drainage is through the splenic vein which joins the portal venous system taking blood into the liver.

11.023 Radiotracers used for evaluating the spleen include all of the following EXCEPT:
   A. 111In labeled WBCs
   B. ^{99m}Tc labeled RBCs, denatured
   C. 111In oxine platelets
   D. ^{99m}Tc sulfur colloid
   E. 201 Tl chloride
   F. ^{99m}Tc albumin colloid

E. is correct.
Spleen specific radiotracers such as heat denatured ^{99m}Tc labeled RBCs, 111In oxine WBCs, and 111In oxine platelets can be used when searching for accessory splenic tissue. 99mTc sulfur colloid or albumin colloid looks at the phagocytic ability of spleen cells.

11.024 In a normal posterior liver-spleen image with ^{99m}Tc labeled colloid, the ratio of the density of the liver to the spleen is approximately:
   A. 1:1
   B. 1:2
   C. 1:3
   D. 2:1

A. is correct.
Normally, the liver and spleen on the posterior view should have the same density (1:1). "Shift of function", where the spleen demonstrates a higher density than the liver may be the result of hepatic damage. In these cases, the bone marrow which is usually not visualized, may be seen on the images as well.

11.025 Bile is produced in the liver and concentrated and stored in the:
   A. duodenum
   B. spleen
   C. gallbladder
   D. pancreas

C. is correct.
The gallbladder stores and concentrates bile which it receives from the common hepatic duct via the cystic duct.

11.026 The right and left hepatic bile ducts join to form the:
   A. cystic duct
   B. gallbladder
   C. common hepatic duct
   D. common bile duct

C. is correct.
The right and left hepatic ducts join to form the common hepatic duct. The cystic duct leads from the gallbladder and joins the common hepatic duct which continues to the duodenum as the common bile duct.

11.027 The gallbladder can hold approximate how many ml of bile?
   A. 10 ml
   B. 50 ml
   C. 100 ml
   D. 150 ml

B. is correct.
The pear-shaped hallow sac about 7-10 cm in length holds about 50 ml of bile. The bile that is secreted by the liver is stored and concentrated in the gallbladder.

11.028 The hormone that is primarily responsible for gallbladder contraction is:
  A. thyroxine
  B. insulin
  C. saliva
  D. cholecystokinin

D. is correct.
Cholecystokinin is secreted into the blood by the duodenum and stimulates gallbladder contraction and the secretion of pancreatic enzymes.

11.029 The nuclear medicine technologist discovers that the patient injected for a biliary scan has had an opioid drug administered for pain previous to coming to the department for the scan. What might be the expected result?
  A. delayed visualization of the gallbladder
  B. delayed visualization of the small bowel
  C. delayed clearance from the common bile duct
  D. all of the above
  E. B and C
  F. none of the above

E. is correct.
The administration of Demerol, morphine, or other opiod drugs induces the contraction of the sphincter of Oddi, resulting in delayed visualization of the small bowel, delayed clearance of the common bile duct, but enhanced visualization of the gallbladder in cases where there is not obstruction of the cystic duct.

11.030 For the evaluation of the gallbladder during hepatobiliary imaging, how long should the patient fast prior to the exam?
  A. 20 minutes
  B. 1 hour
  C. 2-4 hours
  D. 24 hours

C. is correct.
Recent food ingestion may result in gallbladder contraction and a false positive exam. Prolonged fasting (> 24 hours) can also result in a false positive exam if the gallbladder remains full of unlabeled bile. Administration of CCK or fatty meal will cause the gallbladder to contract.

11.031 Hepatobiliary imaging is used in suspected acute cholecystitis to evaluate patency of the cystic duct.
  A. true
  B. false

A. is correct.
Visualization of the gallbladder using radiotracers excludes the diagnosis of acute cholecystitis. Acute cholecystitis is caused by an obstructed cystic duct in 98% of all cases.

11.032 When performing hepatobiliary imaging, the best view to separate the gallbladder activity from activity in the duodenum is the:
  A. left anterior oblique
  B. right anterior oblique
  C. left lateral
  D. right lateral
  E. posterior

A. is correct.
The LAO view will separate the activity in the gallbladder from small intestine. In the anterior position it may be difficult to distinguish activity in the duodenum or right kidney from activity in the gallbladder.

11.033 The most accurate and cost effective study to distinguish nonobstructive versus obstructive jaundice is seen in:
  A. magnetic resonance imaging (MRI)
  B. sonography
  C. ^{99m}Tc IDA imaging
  D. computed tomography (CT)
  E. B and D

B. is correct.
Both CT and ultrasound are more accurate than ^{99m}Tc IDA imaging in nonobstructive vs obstructive jaundice. Because it is highly accurate, non-ionizing, and inexpensive, ultrasound should be the initial diagnostic procedure. CT can be used when ultrasound fails to define the site of the obstruction.

11.034 Indications for hepatobiliary pediatric imaging include:
  A. differentiation between biliary atresia and neonatal hepatitis
  B. evaluation of right upper quadrant masses
  C. evaluation of right upper quadrant pain
  D. all of the above

D. is correct.
Right upper quadrant pain and suspected acute cholecystitis are the primary indications for gallbladder scintigraphy in the adult.

11.035 A congenital dilatation of the extrahepatic biliary tree is known as:
   A. cholangitis
   B. choledochal cyst
   C. choledochojejunostomy
   D. cholestasis

B. is correct.
Choledochal cysts are rare congenital anomalies which usually require surgery to separate the drainage routes for the liver and pancreas.

11.036 Factors which delay the appearance of the gallbladder during hepatobiliary imaging are:
   A. impairment of hepatocyte function
   B. obstruction of the cystic duct
   C. contraction of the gallbladder due to recent food ingestion
   D. obstruction of the biliary ducts proximal to the cystic duct
   E. all of the above
   F. B and D only

E. is correct.
If a study is terminated too early, before 4 hours post injection, the patient may be misdiagnosed as acute cholecystitis when delayed images would show the visualization of the gallbladder. In normal studies, the gallbladder and small bowel are visualized within one hour of injection.

11.037 If the gallbladder is not evident on hepatobiliary imaging by 45 minutes, the technologist should:
   A. terminate the study
   B. continue to take delayed images
   C. have the patient injected with CCK
   D. have the patient ingest a fatty meal and return for images

B. is correct.
In acute cholecystitis, the gallbladder will not visualize at 60 minutes nor on delays up to 4 hours post-injection. In chronic cholecystitis, the gallbladder visualization will be delayed between 2-4 hours post-injection.

11.038 ^{99m}Tc IDAs concentrate in:
   A. hepatocytes
   B. lymphocytes
   C. erythrocytes
   D. all of the above

A. is correct.
The hepatocytes clear the IDA labeled materials from the blood in a mechanism similar to the transport mechanism of bilirubin. This makes these agents specific for liver tissue.

SECTION 12: CENTRAL NERVOUS SYSTEM SCINTIGRAPHY

TUTORIAL

The central nervous system (CNS) consists of the brain and spinal cord which primarily interpret incoming sensory information and respond based on past experiences. The two cerebral hemispheres are the most superior portion of the brain and are divided into four lobes; frontal, temporal, parietal, and occipital. The primary motor area occupies the posterior portion of the frontal lobe and is responsible for conscious or voluntary movement. Impulses traveling form the body's sensory receptors (such as pain, pressure, heat and cold) are localized in the area of the parietal lobes. The temporal lobe is responsible for hearing and language organization, and the occipital lobe is specialized for vision.

Most of the cerebral tissue, the deeper white matter, is composed of fiber tracts carrying impulses to or from the cortex, or the outermost gray matter portion of the cerebrum. Gray matter masses within the cerebral hemispheres called the basal ganglia relay messages to the cerebral cortex. The thalamus consists of two large lobes of gray matter that act as a relay station for sensory impulses passing up to the cortex for interpretation. The hypothalamus and the hypophysis (pituitary gland) are important in the regulation of many feedback systems including the hypothalamus-pituitary-thyroid axis. The cerebellum in the posterior fossa of the skull controls orientation in space.

Most conventional brain scanning has been based on the concept and functional characteristics of the intact blood brain barrier (BBB). The blood brain barrier is not impermeable, but merely selective. Large molecules such as plasma proteins and many toxins are excluded from entering the brain parenchyma. Lipid soluble substances can pass through passively as a result of a concentration gradient between the blood and the brain.

Conventional brain scanning was really "non-brain" scanning. Gamma emitting radiopharmaceuticals would only enter the brain if the blood brain barrier was broken down and accumulation occurred as a result of the increased permeability. Radiopharmaceuticals that are used include ^{99m}Tc DTPA and GH. ^{99m}Tc pertechnatate is the <u>least</u> desirable because of the need to administer potassium perchlorate to block the activity in the choroid plexus. Currently there are radiopharmaceuticals that have the characteristics needed for metabolic brain imaging; BBB permeability, retention in the brain parenchyma, and can be labeled with gamma emitters that can be imaged easily. 123I iodoamphetamine (IMP) and 123I (HIPDM) and ^{99m}Tc -d,1-hexamethyl propylene amine oxime (HMPAO or Ceretec) and ^{99m}Tc-oxo-1,1-N,N'-ethylenediylbis-d,d-cysteinediethyl ester (^{99m}Tc-ECD) cross the intact blood brain barrier and distribute in the cerebral cortex relative to the regional cerebral blood flow.

The relationship of planar brain imaging, PET, and SPECT and the clinical utility of each has been established.

12.001 Radiopharmaceuticals are normally excluded from brain tissue due to an intact:
   A. blood brain barrier
   B. neurologic impairment
   C. systemic circulatory system
   D. cerebral ventricular system

A. is correct.
The blood-brain barrier is a network of capillaries in the brain with a nearly impenetrable barrier to shield the brain from toxins in the blood stream and biochemical fluctuations.

12.002 The blood- brain barrier is:
   A. composed of four cell layers
   B. visible on all brain images
   C. responsible for active tumor growth
   D. an anatomic and physiological concept

D. is correct.
The tightly packed cells lining the blood vessels in the brain form a physiological barrier to shield the delicate brain tissue, but permit nutrients to cross the barrier.

12.003 During planar brain imaging using radiopharmaceuticals that do not penetrate the intact blood-brain barrier , the "crescent sign" is highly suggestive of what condition?
   A. CVA
   B. skull fractures
   C. metastases
   D. subdural hematoma

D. is correct.
Chronic subdural hematoma will concentrate a radiopharmaceutical between the dura mater and arachnoid membrane of the brain, where the collection of fluid is compressing brain tissue giving a crescent moon appearance on the scan. The cerebral radionuclide angiogram will show a peripheral photon-deficient concavity.

12.004 During planar brain imaging using radiopharmaceuticals that do not penetrate the intact blood-brain barrier, the "doughnut sign" may be indicative of:
   A. a tumor with central necrosis
   B. an abscess
   C. a hematoma
   D. all of the above

D. is correct.
The doughnut sign is a ring of increased activity surrounding a photopenic or "cold" area. All of the above conditions could demonstrate this appearance on a scan.

12.005 The venous phase of a perfusion study is marked by:
   A. the arrival of activity in the superior sagittal sinus
   B. internal carotid artery activity
   C. a vascular blush over the cerebral hemispheres
   D. the arrival of activity in the middle cerebral arteries

A. is correct.
The arrival of activity in the superior sagittal sinus marks the beginning of the venous phase of cerebral perfusion; the sinuses drain through the internal jugular veins.

12.006 The spinal cord is on average between 16 - 18 inches in length and extends from the foramen magnum to the sacral spine.
   A. true
   B. false

B. is correct.
The spinal cord ends at the conus medularis at T12 - L1 and does not extend into the sacral spine.

12.007 CSF (cerebral spinal fluid) circulates in the _____ space.
   A. subarachnoid
   B. subdural
   C. interstitial
   D. epidural

A. is correct.
The sub arachnoid space lies between the arachnoid membrane and the pia mater of the brain and spinal cord and provides a pathway for the flow of CSF to reabsorption by the arachnoid villi in the superior sagittal sinus.

12.008 The normal appearance of cerebral spinal fluid is:
   A. yellow
   B. cloudy
   C. clear and colorless
   D. pink or red tinged
   E. all of the above

C. is correct.
Disease, infection, injury, may alter the appearance of the CSF which is normally clear and colorless.

12.009 Normal CSF imaging protocols demonstrate the visualization of the radiotracer within the ventricles at:
   A. 6 hours
   B. 24 hours
   C. 48 hours
   D. 96 hours
   E. none of the above

E. is correct.
Normal ventricular function will not accumulate activity within the ventricles.

12.010 Which of the following most likely affects the rate of flow of CSF?
   A. gender
   B. age
   C. body position
   D. height
   E. none of the above

B. is correct.
Elderly patients may demonstrate slower rates of CSF flow when compared to younger patients. The time required from CSF production in the choroid plexes to reabsorption is 6 to 36 hours.

12.011 Neurotransmission is dependent upon the presence of _____ to provide the energy (ATP), required for proper functioning.
   A. potassium
   B. oxygen
   C. glucose
   D. all of the above
   E. B and C only

E. is correct.
Ninety-five percent of the energy required for normal brain function results from the oxidation of glucose. The brain is one of the largest consumers of energy in the body.

12.012 When performing a brain scan using ^{99m}Tc pertechnatate, a technologist notes that the patient had a previous bone scan within 24 hours. What might be the result of the current brain scan?
   A. may be a false positive
   B. may be a false negative
   C. the choroid plexus will show
   D. the increase background will make the scan unreadable

B. is correct.
If there is residual stannous ion, the ^{99m}Tc pertechnatate will bind to the red blood cells and not be available to bind with the intracerebral lesions that may be present giving a false negative result.

12.013 In cerebral radionuclide angiography, the scintillation camera should be started _____ after the injection of the radiopharmaceutical.
   A. immediately
   B. 12-15
   C. 20-25 seconds
   D. 30-35 seconds
   E. one minute

A. is correct.
Imaging should begin when activity is seen on the persistence scope or monitor or immediately after injection. The appearance of radiopharmaceutical is generally seen within 5-10 seconds after a successful bolus injection.

12.014 Static brain images should be positioned to include as much facial activity as possible.
   A. true
   B. false

B. is correct.
Reducing the amount of facial activity in the static views will provide increased counting statistics from the area of interest.

12.015 Which of the following central nervous system studies is routinely used for the determination of brain death?
   A. a blood brain barrier study using ^{99m}Tc DTPA
   B. a cisternogram using 111In DTPA
   C. a cerebral arteriogram using ^{99m}Tc MAA
   D. all are routinely used

A. is correct.
Perfusion, blood pool, and delayed images may be acquired. Computer generated time-activity curves and quantitative analysis may be performed with the appropriate software.

12.016 Which of the following radiopharmaceuticals is NOT based on detecting a compromised blood-brain barrier?
A. ^{99m}Tc pertechnatate
B. ^{99m}Tc DTPA
C. ^{99m}Tc GH
D. 201 Tl
E. ^{99m}Tc HMPAO

E. is correct.
^{99m}Tc HMPAO crosses the blood-brain barrier and can be used to reflect region blood flow as it is trapped in the brain proportional to the cerebral blood flow.

12.017 A disadvantage associated with imaging with ^{99m}Tc HMPAO is that:
A. it has a long retention time
B. physical characteristics are inferior to other imaging agents
C. it is unstable and must be administered within 30 minutes of preparation
D. the physiological distribution is dependent upon the CSF flow

C. is correct.
^{99m}Tc HMPAO is unstable in aqueous solution and must be administered within 30 minutes of preparation. Many departments wait until the arrival of the patient into the department to prepare the radiopharmaceutical for injection.

12.018 Which statement regarding ^{99m}Tc HMPAO is FALSE?
A. it concentrates in metabolically active brain cells
B. uptake is predominately in the white matter
C. it can be used in the evaluation of CVA
D. it crosses the blood brain barrier

B. is correct.
Uptake of the SPECT perfusion imaging radiopharmaceuticals distributes relative to the regional cerebral blood flow which is more predominate in the gray matter areas of the brain; primarily the cerebral cortex and basal ganglia.

12.019 When preparing to scan a patient to be injected with a perfusion SPECT radiopharmaceutical, it is a good idea to:
A. leave the room lights on to keep the patient alert
B. dim the lights and let the patient relax
C. immobilize the patient's head
D. position the camera far enough from the patient's head so that the camera will not frighten him/her
E. A, C, and D
F. B and C only

F. is correct.
In order to minimize the effect from environmental stimuli, the imaging room should be quiet and dimly lit, an IV line should be in place so there is no stimulation from the pain of the injection, the detector should be positioned as close to the patient's head as possible for optimal resolution, and the head should be secured to prevent rotation or movement during the examination. It is advisable to stay in the room with the patient throughout the procedure to insure that no movement occurs.

12.020 Indications for SPECT perfusion imaging include all of the following EXCEPT:
A. evaluation of cerebrovascular diseases
B. pituitary microadenoma
C. localization of seizure foci
D. evaluation of head trauma

B. is correct.
The strength of SPECT perfusion imaging lies in the ability to evaluate regional cerebral blood flow and the pathologies associated with the interruption of that flow. The size and location of the pituitary gland make it difficult to resolve pathology using SPECT perfusion imaging.

12.021 Some considerations for possible errors that could contribute to an undiagnostic scan include:
A. patient comfort and immobility for the duration of the study
B. patient to detector distance
C. environmental stimuli during the injection
D. artifacts from poor quality control technical factors
E. all of the above

E. is correct.
Quality control of the tomographic system will reduce artifacts, evaluation of the patient's condition and ability to hold still for a specific length of time will reduce motion artifacts, using a table with a cephalic extension for the patient's head will allow closer detector distance, and maintaining a quiet environment will reduce the possibility of the distribution being affected by external stimuli.

12.022 The usual average dose for ^{99m}Tc-labeled SPECT perfusion imaging agents such as HMPAO (Ceretec) and ECD (Neurolite) is:
  A. 3-5 mCi (111 -185 MBq)
  B. 5-10 mCi (185-370 MBq)
  C. 15 mCi (555MBq)
  D. 20 mCi (740 MBq)

D is correct.
The average dose for the rCBF (regional cerebral blood flow) radiopharmaceuticals using ^{99m}Tc, is 20 mCi (740 MBq).

12.023 The usual average dose for 123I-labeled SPECT perfusion imaging agents such as IMP and its analog HIPDM is:
  A. 1-2 mCi (37-74 MBq)
  B. 3-6 mCi (111-222 MBq)
  C. 10 mCi (370 MBq)
  D. 15 mCi (555MBq)

B. is correct.
The average dose for the 123I -labeled radiopharmaceuticals is 3-6 mCi. Lugol's solution (3 drops) may be given 3 hours prior to injection to block thyroid uptake of radioiodine.

12.024 The radiopharmaceutical used for assessment of CSF dynamics is administered:
  A. intravenously
  B. subcutaneously
  C. intrathecally
  D. intramuscularly
  E. intradermally

C. is correct.
A lumbar puncture is performed (at the level of L3-L4 or L4-L5) and the radiopharmaceutical is administered intrathecally or within the spinal canal (literally, within a sheath).

12.025 The radiopharmaceutical most often used for CSF imaging is:
  A. ^{99m}Tc tagged red cells
  B. 111In DTPA
  C. 201 Tl chloride
  D. 67 Ga citrate

B. is correct.
111In DTPA has the least chemical toxicity, a half-life that allows for adequate imaging through the length of the study (T1/2 = 2.8 days), a desirable energy for imaging (173 and 247 keV), low radiation dose to the patient, and it follows the physiology of CSF flow.

12.026 The most common clinical indication(s) for cisternography (or CSF imaging) include(s):
  A. Alzheimer's disease
  B. schizophrenia
  C. normal pressure hydrocephalus (NPH)
  D. headache

C. is correct.
Evaluation of normal pressure hydrocephalus is the most common clinical indication. Identification of cerebrospinal fluid (CSF) leaks is also an indication for performing the examination.

12.027 The usual dose of 111In DTPA for CSF imaging is in the range of _____ 111In DTPA.
  A. 250 - 300 uCi
  B. 500 uCi - 1 mCi
  C. 1 mCi -1.5 mCi
  D. 2 mCi - 2.5 mCi

B. is correct.
The usual dose for adults for CSF imaging is 500 uCi (18.5 MBq) to 1 mCi (37 MBq) of 111In DTPA via intrathecal injection.

12.028 In order to rule out extravasation of the injected dose, what should be done?
  A. the patient should be position with his/her head lower than his/her feet
  B. imaging of the injection site should be done immediately
  C. imaging of the head and neck should be done immediately
  D. flow images with the camera positioned over the patient's head should be taken

B. is correct.
In order to rule out extravasation of the radiopharmaceutical outside of the subarachnoid space, the injection site should be imaged immediately. A thin narrow band of activity and appearance of tracer in the basal cisterns at 2-3 hours post injection would indicate a successful injection.

12.029 What should be done to determine the diagnosis of CSF leaks such as in rhinorrhea and otorrhea?
  A. absorbent pledgets are placed in the area suspected of leakage
  B. images at 24 hours should be taken of the suspected area
  C. images of the basal cisterns should be taken
  D. a vertex view should be taken

A. is correct.
A physician should place a pledget in the suspected area and a heparinized blood sample taken from the patient. Normal pledget to plasma ratios are 1:1.3.

12.030 The purpose of taking blood samples from a patient suspected of a CSF leak is to:
  A. establish a baseline hematocrit
  B. determine slow CSF flow
  C. determine subarachnoid space blockage
  D. establish a baseline plasma count

D. is correct.
Pledgets and plasma are counted and results are expressed as a ratio of pledget activity (cpm) over plasma activity (cpm). Activity that is 3 to 4 times that of background (plasma) indicates a significant leak.

12.031 If a technologist injects a patient with 1 mCi (37 MBq) of ^{99m}Tc DTPA, intravenously, for a ventricular shunt study, the administration of the radiopharmaceutical is:
  A. correct dose, correct radiopharmaceutical, correct route of administration
  B. correct dose, incorrect radiopharmaceutical, correct route of administration
  C. correct dose, correct radiopharmaceutical, incorrect route of administration
  D. incorrect dose, correct radiopharmaceutical, incorrect route of administration

C. is correct.
According to NRC regulations, this would be a misadministration. The route of administration is other than what is intended by the prescribing physician. Ventricular shunt studies are performed using 1 mCi of ^{99m}Tc DTPA in a small volume (less than 0.1 mL) and is injected into the shunt reservoir by the neurosurgeon or nuclear medicine physician.

SECTION 13: INFREQUENT PROCEDURES

TUTORIAL

There are many procedures that are performed in the nuclear medicine department less often than the more common procedures such as skeletal, cardiac, lung, thyroid, and renal scans. However they provide valuable information and may take the place of a more invasive diagnostic procedure.

Included are the gastrointestinal studies such as salivary gland imaging, gastric emptying studies, gastroesophageal reflux, esophageal transit or motility studies, Meckel's diverticulum detection, and gastrointestinal bleeding site localization. Some of these studies take advantage of the biorouting of ^{99m}Tc pertechnetate to the gastric mucosa and salivary glands, while others involve the ingestion of a radiolabeled food to examine the function of the GI tract. By tagging red blood cells with ^{99m}Tc pertechnetate, one can localize active bleeding sites in the bowel.

Lymphoscintigraphy provides a way to examine the lymph chains for staging of Hodgkin's disease and other diseases that involve the lymph nodes. This study can be invaluable in preoperative evaluation of lymph nodes for metastases or radiation therapy.

A dacrocystogram is performed to determine the patentcy of the lacrimal duct and is less invasive than the radiographic contrast study.

Tumor imaging with 67 Ga has been widely used in the past for a few types of cancer for which the malignant tissue has an affinity for 67 Ga. Studies done using 201Tl and ^{99m}Tc sestimibi in localizing malignant breast tissue and metastatic sites, and in finding malignant brain tumors with functional tissue following radiation therapy have been successful and provide the diagnostician with information that may not be available through any other imaging modality.

Parathyroid imaging provides the surgeon with the localization of parathyroid adenomas and is especially sensitive when combined with computer subtraction methods. Imaging of the adrenal glands in nuclear medicine is interesting because of the two distinctly different functions of the adrenal tissue. The adrenal cortical pathophysiology which involve hormones derived from cholesterol, are imaged with radiotracers such as 131 I NP-59 (a iodinated cholesterol analog), while the adrenal medulla utilizes 131 I mIBG scintigraphy to localize pheochromocytoma.

Venography, shunt imaging, and monoclonal antibodies (for ovarian and colorectal cancer) are briefly included in this chapter as well.

13.001 The radiopharmaceutical of choice for Salivary Gland Imaging is:
   A. ^{99m}Tc DTPA
   B. ^{99m}Tc Pertechnetate
   C. 131I -Sodium Iodide
   D. 123I-Sodium Iodide

B. is correct.
^{99m}Tc Pertechnetate is localized in gastric mucosa as well as functioning cells in the parotid, salivary, and thyroid glands.

13.002 Salivary Gland Imaging with stimulation can usually be completed in approximately:
   A. 30 min.
   B. 1 hr.
   C. 2 hr.
   D. 4 hr.

B. is correct.
1 hr. Typically, images are taken at 2, 5, 10, 15, 20, and 30 min post-injection. After images are checked, the salivary glands are stimulated for 10-15 min. Post-stimulation views are then obtained.

13.003 A patient's salivary glands may be stimulated with each of the following EXCEPT
   A. gum
   B. lemon juice
   C. water
   D. perchlorate

C. is correct.
Water; all others stimulate secretion of saliva in the glands.

13.004 Images of a patient with Sjogren's Syndrome typically show:
   A. Decreased activity is salivary tissue with patchy decrease in concentration.
   B. increased concentration
   C. smooth and round lesions with an absence of activity
   D. normal uptake in salivary glands

A. is correct.
Decreased activity in salivary tissues with patchy decrease in concentration is the typical appearance for Sjogrens's Syndrome.

13.005 The glands normally visualized on a salivary gland scan include:
   A. salivary glands
   B. parotid glands
   C. thyroid gland
   D. all of the above
   E. A and B only

D. is correct.
^{99m}Tc pertechnetate is taken up by the salivary, parotid, and thyroid glands and all should be included in the field of view

13.006 A salivary gland scan reveals a focal area of increased concentration of ^{99m}Tc pertechnetate within a salivary gland. This is most likely a(n):
   A. abscess
   B. cyst
   C. Warthin's tumor
   D. metastatic lesion

C. is correct.
Warthin's tumor; others may show decreased concentration of radiotracer.

13.007 In a patient with normal thyroid function, the activity in the salivary gland is _____the activity in the thyroid gland.
   A. greater than
   B. less than
   C. equal to

C. is correct.
Equal to; this is a relative assessment; can be done visually on film or quantitatively by computer.

13.008 When positioning a patient for a salivary gland scan, which landmark should be placed at the bottom of a SFOV?

    A. nose
    B. chin
    C. suprasternal notch
    D. xyphoid

C. is correct.
Suprasternal notch; this will allow you to include the thyroid, salivary and parotid glands in the image.

13.009 Radiopharmaceuticals for lymph node imaging are injected:

    A. intravenously
    B. intrathecally
    C. intramuscularly
    D. subcutaneously

D. is correct.
subcutaneously to allow access into the lymph node system.

13.010 Important factors to consider when preparing the radiopharmaceutical for lymph node imaging include all of the following EXCEPT:

    A. temperature
    B. particle size
    C. dose
    D. volume to be injected

A. is correct.
Temperature; Lymph node imaging is performed using ^{99m}Tc Sulfur Colloid (particle size between 0.2 and 0.5 micron), 0.5 to 1.0 mCi (18.5 to 37 MBq) in a volume not to exceed 0.25 ml per injection site.

13.011 To visualize the axillary and apical lymph node chains, the proper injection site would be:

    A. dorsum of the processes mastoideus
    B. medial two interdigital webs of the feet
    C. posterior rectus sheath below the rib cage
    D. medial two interdigital webs of the hands

D. is correct.
The medial two interdigital webs of the hands would allow the visualization of the axillary and apical nodal chains.

13.012 When interpreting a lymphoscintogram, the evaluation is based on which of the following criteria?

    A. the continuity of the lymphatic chain
    B. the width of the radioactive chain
    C. the intensity of the uptake
    D. the topographic distribution of the radioactivity
    E. the radioactivity within the liver
    F. all of the above
    G. A and C only

F. is correct.
Attention must be given to any interruption, enlargement, displacement, or collateral circulation involving the lymph node chain. Since a radioactive colloid is used, it should travel to the liver if the lymph node chain is patent.

13.013 The physician instructs you to position the patient to visualize the cervical nodes. You should position the camera over the patient's:

    A. neck
    B. chest
    C. pelvis
    D. head

A. is correct.
Neck; the radioactivity can be seen as far as the supraclavicular region.

13.014 The most important factor for lymphatic transport is:

    A. compression of lymphatic vessels via peristalsis
    B. patient position
    C. blood flow in vessels parallel to lymphatic vessels
    D. compression of lymphatic vessels by muscular contraction

D. is correct.
Compression of lymphatic vessels by muscular contraction distributes the injected radiocolloids.

13.015 The correct collimator used in dacrocystography is:
A. converging
B. pinhole with 2mm insert
C. low energy high resolution
D. low energy high sensitivity

B. is correct.
Pinhole with 2mm insert provides the best resolution for imaging

13.016 The typical dose of ^{99m}Tc Pertechnetate delivered per eye in a dacrocystogram is:
A. 50 uCi (1.85 MBq)
B. 200 uCi (7.4 MBq)
C. 500 uCi (18.5 MBq)
D. 1.0 mCi (37 MBq)

B. is correct.
200 uCi (7.4 MBq) of ^{99m}Tc Pertechnetate. This can be done using 10 drops of a solution prepared by diluting 10 mCi (370 MBq) of ^{99m}Tc Pertechnetate to 0.5 ml with normal saline.

13.017 A normal dacrocystogram is interpreted by:
A. activity in the area of the nose in 10 - 15 min
B. accumulation of activity in the nasal lacrimal duct
C. activity in the area of the nose in 20 - 30 min
D. it depends on the position of the patient

A. is correct.
A normal scan produces activity in the area of the nose in 10 - 15 min

13.018 The portion of the stomach which is located at the distal end of the esophagus is known as the:
A. fundus
B. body
C. pylorus
D. curvature

A. is correct.
The upper part of the stomach at the junction of the esophagus is called the cardia, which dilates into the fundus of the stomach. The next parts of the stomach are the body, antrum, and pylorus which is at the end joining the duodenum.

13.019 Below is a list of radiolabeled meals used in the determination of solid gastric emptying time. Which is considered the most stable product?
A. surface in vitro chicken liver
B. injected in vitro chicken liver
C. in vivo labeled chicken liver
D. sulfur colloid egg
E. macroaggregated albumin egg

C. is correct.
This is a stable intracellular label to the liver parenchymal tissue.

13.020 A dual isotope gastric emptying study is performed using ^{99m}Tc Sulfur Colloid and 111In DTPA. The correct window setting(s) is(are):
A. 140 keV 20%
B. 173 keV 20%
C. 247 keV 20%
D. A and B
E. A and C
F. B and C

D. is correct.
The 173 keV photon is the more abundant of the two 111In peaks.

13.021 Which pathology listed below is NOT a cause of delayed gastric emptying?
A. scleroderma
B. hyperthyroidism
C. peptic ulceration
D. diabetes mellitus
E. vagotomy

B. is correct.
Abnormal gastric emptying results from a mechanical or functional disorder. All of the above, with the exception of hyperthyroidism, can cause delayed emptying. Hyperthyroidism may result in rapid gastric emptying.

13.022 All of the statements listed below are true EXCEPT:
  A. liquid meals empty faster than solid meals
  B. liquids may accelerate the emptying of solids
  C. solid emptying is accelerated in the presence of fats
  D. gastric emptying is affected by many factors including volume, caloric and nutrient content, and pH.

C. is correct.
Fats will slow the emptying process.

13.023 The gastric emptying rate of liquids can best be described as:
  A. linear
  B. exponential
  C. delayed
  D. accelerate

B. is correct.
Liquids empty faster than solids and produce an exponentially shaped curve.

13.024 The gastric emptying rate of solids can be described as:
  A. linear
  B. exponential
  C. delayed
  D. accelerated

A. is correct.
Solids produce a linearly shaped curve.

13.025 A patient should be NPO at least 4 hours prior to which of the following studies?
  A. Meckel's scan
  B. gastric emptying
  C. GI bleed
  D. salivary gland
  E. all of the above
  F. A and B only

F. is correct.
In the case of gastric emptying, having the patient NPO from midnight on is recommended. It is important not to have interference from any conditions that would affect either gastric motility or in the case of a Meckel's scan, the uptake of the radiotracer by ectopic gastric mucosa.

13.026 Normal solid gastric emptying half-times should be determined at each laboratory. From the choices below, which time is reported frequently in the literature as a normal solid emptying half-time?
  A. 30 - 60 min
  B. 60 - 90 min
  C. 100 - 150 min
  D. 150 - 200 min

B. is correct.
Normal half-times have been reported between 45 min. and greater than 2 hours.

13.027 The most common indication for performing a pediatric gastroesophageal reflux study is:
  A. gastroparesis
  B. abdominal pain
  C. chronic respiratory problems
  D. frequent vomiting

C. is correct.
Aspiration of gastric contents has been implicated in patients with recurrent pneumonias or asthma.

13.028 The recommended minimum dosage of ^{99m}Tc Sulfur Colloid for a pediatric gastroesophageal reflux study is:
  A. 50 uCi (1.85 MBq)
  B. 150 uCi (5.55 MBq)
  C. 300 uCi (11.1 MBq)
  D. 500 uCi (18.5 MBq)

B. is correct.
The maximum dose is 1 mCi (37 MBq) of ^{99m}Tc Sulfur Colloid added to the normal volume of milk or formula for that patient. The final concentration is approximately 5 uCi (.185 MBq)/ml.

13.029 Symptoms of gastroesophageal reflux include:
   A. regurgitation
   B. epigastric discomfort
   C. pyrosis
   D. all of the above

D. is correct.
Indications for the gastroesophageal reflux scintigram include symptoms of reflux esophagitis (epigastric or chest pain and regurgitation), and pyrosis or heartburn.

13.030 The normal patient undergoing a gastroesophageal reflux examination would demonstrate _____ with an increase of mechanical abdominal pressure.
   A. no reflux
   B. spontaneous reflux
   C. delayed reflux
   D. induced reflux

A. is correct.
The increase in abdominal pressure is useful in detecting subtle cases of reflux. The digital computerized image and counts can be used to calculate the reflux index.

13.031 A pediatric gastroesophageal reflux study can safely be terminated at what time?
   A. 1 hr
   B. 2 hrs
   C. 8 hrs
   D. 24 hrs

D. is correct.
Static anterior and posterior images of the lungs should be obtained intermittently over a 24 hr period to look for evidence of aspiration.

13.032 What additional maneuvers can be used to augment gastroesophageal reflux?
   A. pharmacologic intervention
   B. imaging continuously for 60 min
   C. abdominal binder with sphygmomanometer
   D. imaging during the swallowing phase

C. is correct.
The abdominal pressure generated by the binder is helpful in bringing out subtle cases of reflux; it is believed to simulate the pressure at the GE junction that is comparable to that developed when bending over or performing a Valsalva maneuver. May want to be avoided in infants and after recent abdominal surgery.

13.033 Normally the lining of the esophagus consists of stratified squamous epithelium; however in patients with chronic gastroesophageal reflux, the esophageal mucosa is changed into columnar epithelium, identical to that found in the stomach. The abnormality is termed:
   A. esophagitis
   B. Zenker's diverticulum
   C. hiatal hernia
   D. Barrett's esophagus

D. is correct.
Barrett's esophagus; Columnar epithelium located in the esophagus is prone to peptic ulcer and stricture. These patients also have an increased risk of adenocarcinoma of the esophagus.

13.034 When using an abdominal binder, the binder should be placed:
   A. at the level of the xyphoid
   B. above the iliac crests
   C. below the rib margin
   D. at the level of the umbilicus

C. is correct.
Place the binder below the level of the ribs to prevent rib fracture.

13.035 The preferred radiopharmaceutical used in LeVeen Shunt imaging is:
   A. ^{99m}Tc MAA
   B. ^{99m}Tc DTPA
   C. ^{99m}Tc Sulfur Colloid
   D. ^{99m}Tc Pertechnetate

A. is correct.
^{99m}Tc MAA; it is possible to use ^{99m}Tc Sulfur Colloid, however this may cause confusion in interpretation if there is difficulty in separating the liver from the ascites.

13.036 A LeVeen Shunt imaging procedure using 3 mCi
(111 MBq) of ^{99m}Tc MAA is complete when:
- A. the tubing is visualized
- B. the lungs are visualized
- C. the liver is visualized
- D. there is homogeneous activity throughout the abdomen

B. is correct.
A normal lung image indicates normal return of the ^{99m}Tc MAA from the LeVeen Shunt into the venous system.

13.037 Which radiopharmaceutical(s) listed below has been found extremely useful in locating malignant breast tumors?
- A. 210 Tl chloride
- B. 67 Ga citrate
- C. ^{99m}Tc Sestimibi
- D. A and B
- E. A and C
- F. none of the above

E. is correct.
Thallium 201 and Technetium ^{99m}Tc Sestimibi have been extremely useful in patients with dense or dysplastic breast tissue. These radionuclides are also useful in detecting malignant brain tumors.

13.038 Detection of a Meckel's diverticulum is possible with ^{99m}Tc pertechnatate since it localizes in the:
- A. salivary glands
- B. gastric mucosa
- C. choroid plexus
- D. thyroid gland

B. is correct.
The localization will occur only in those diverticula that contain ectopic gastric mucosal cells.

13.039 The usual location of a Meckel's diverticulum is in the:
- A. stomach
- B. esophagus
- C. ileum
- D. colon

C. is correct.
The diverticulum lies proximal to the ileocecal valve and may contain tissues representing ileal mucosa as well as gastric, duodenal, pancreas and colon.

13.040 The increase in activity with time that occurs in the Meckel's diverticulum parallels the increasing activity of the:
- A. kidney
- B. stomach
- C. bladder
- D. liver

B. is correct.
the increase inactivity reflects the accumulation of activity in the gastric mucosal cells.

13.041 Typically, a Meckel's diverticula will appear as a focal "hot" spot located in the:
- A. right upper quadrant
- B. left upper quadrant
- C. right lower quadrant
- D. left lower quadrant

C. is correct.
Right lower quadrant in the location of the ileum, proximal to the ileocecal valve.

13.042 Pharmacologic intervention with Meckel's diverticulum imaging can include all of the following EXCEPT:
- A. glucagon
- B. pentagastrin
- C. cholecystokinin
- D. cimetidine

C. is correct.
Glucagon will promote pooling and prevent the downstream wash of pertechnatate; pentagastrin has been shown to increase the uptake of pertechnatate; and cimetidine blocks secretion of pertechnatate from gastric mucosa, improving the target to background ratio.

13.043 A Meckel's diverticulum is most likely to be found in a patient:
  A. under the age of 2
  B. between the ages of 12 and 20
  C. over the age of 35
  D. none of the above

A. is correct.
It is possible to find a Meckel's diverticulum in any of these age groups, but the most common is under the age of 2.

13.044 The standard adult dose of ^{99m}Tc pertechnatate for a Meckel's scan is:
  A. 5 mCi (185 MBq)
  B. 10 mCi (370 MBq)
  C. 15 mCi (555 MBq)
  D. 20 mCi (740 MBq)

B. is correct.

13.045 Patient preparation for GI blood loss imaging procedures includes:
  A. 2 hour fast
  B. 12 hour fast
  C. cleansing enemas
  D. none of the above

D. is correct.
There is no patient preparation needed and imaging can be accomplished during the time of active bleeding.

13.046 Localization of a GI bleed is difficult by radionuclide imaging methods because:
  A. only sites of active bleeding are visualized
  B. the amount of bleeding can be too small to be seen
  C. the bleeding site may be masked by surrounding activity
  D. all of the above

D. is correct.
Delayed imaging may assist in localizing intermittent bleeds; computer acquisition may be useful in subtle bleeds and in determining the transit of activity through the bowel.

13.047 ^{99m}Tc Sulfur Colloid used in gastrointestinal bleeding imaging is in the amount of:
  A. 0 -5 mCi (0-185 MBq)
  B. 5-10 mCi (185-370 MBq)
  C. 10 - 15 mCi (370 - 555 MBq)
  D. 15 - 20 mCi (555 - 740 MBq)

C. is correct.
A dose two to three times higher than used in liver scanning is used to image active bleeding sites.

13.048 Using ^{99m}Tc sulfur Colloid to diagnose a gastrointestinal bleed, imaging can safely be terminated at 30-60 min because:
  A. the liver and spleen activity is too intense
  B. the tag begins to break down
  C. sulfur colloid does not remain in circulation
  D. interference by bladder activity

C. is correct.
Sulfur colloid is phagocytized by RES cells and does not remain in circulation.

13.049 Activity seen in the area of the bowel at 24 hrs on a ^{99m}Tc labeled RBC GI Bleeding study is indicative of:
  A. a positive study
  B. questionable because it may not be at the actual bleeding site
  C. due to breakdown of the tag
  D. all of the above
  E. B and C

E. is correct.
It may be due to bleeding, however peristalsis will have moved the blood from the actual bleeding site, and unless you can document movement of the blood, free pertechnatate due to loss of the tag is also a valid explanation.

13.050 To evaluate an active upper gastrointestinal bleed, the radiopharmaceutical of choice would be:
- A. ^{99m}Tc Sulfur Colloid
- B. ^{99m}Tc Labeled RBCs
- C. neither of the above

B. is correct.
Normal liver and spleen uptake by ^{99m}Tc Sulfur Colloid would interfere with detecting an upper GI bleed.

13.051 An ultrasound examination demonstrates an incidental liver mass. The patient is referred for a 3-phase liver scan using ^{99m}Tc labeled RBCs. The results reveal an area of hypoperfusion and increased delayed blood pool images. This pattern is indicative of:
- A. hepatoma
- B. cyst
- C. cavernous hemangioma
- D. metastases

C. is correct.
Cavernous hemangioma is the most common benign liver tumor, characterized by decreased blood flow due to the abnormal vessels, with blood pool images which show increasing uptake over time.

13.052 GI Bleed scanning with ^{99m}Tc labeled RBCs is most useful in patients with:
- A. severe lower GI hemorrhage
- B. occult bleeding
- C. active but not immediately life threatening bleeding
- D. chronic lower GI blood loss

C. is correct.
Active but not immediately life threatening blood loss; because of the potential length of the examination.

13.053 An area of expanded blood pool is noted on a GI bleeding scan using ^{99m}Tc labeled RBCs. It is located in the center of the abdomen and maintains its relationship to the aorta on an LAO view. This activity is most likely due to:
- A. an active bleed
- B. aortic aneurysm
- C. inflammatory bowel disease
- D. small bowel bleeding

B. is correct.
An active bleed is documented by movement of the blood through the bowel. Activity which remains unchanged is most likely due to some other cause.

13.054 A computer technique which may be useful in diagnosing an active GI bleed is:
- A. background subtraction
- B. SPECT imaging
- C. cinematic display
- D. ROI analysis

C. is correct.
Cinematic display may be useful in visualizing the movement or non-movement of an area of interest.

13.055 A patient is suspected of having CSF rhinorrhea. Special imaging considerations include:
- A. imaging the patient upright to prevent CSF leakage
- B. placing cotton pledgets into the nasal cavity
- C. placing pledgets into the ear canal
- D. drawing blood plasma samples
- E. all of the above
- F. B and C
- G. B and D
- H. C and D

G. is correct.
Placing cotton pledgets into the nasal cavity and comparing the activity on the pledgets to that found in the blood plasma.

13.056 A patient with CSF rhinnorhea will produce pledget activity:
- A. less than blood plasma activity
- B. equal to blood plasma activity
- C. greater than blood plasma activity

C. is correct.
Normal pledget activity will be less than or equal to blood plasma activity.

13.057 Which radiopharmaceutical listed below would be the best choice for determination of ventricular shunt patency?
A. 111 In DTPA
B. ^{99m}Tc DTPA
C. ^{99m}Tc MAA
D. ^{99m}Tc pertechnatate

B. is correct.
^{99m}Tc DTPA will demonstrate shunt patency and be excreted from the body via the kidneys without excessive radiation dose or blood background.

13.058 The usual number and location of parathyroid glands is:
A. 3; anterior and superior to the thyroid gland
B. 3; posterior and superior to the thyroid gland
C. 4; posterior and superior to the thyroid gland
D. 4; posterior and inferior to the thyroid gland
E. 4; embedded in the thyroid gland

D. is correct.
The usual number of parathyroid glands is 4; two superior and 2 inferior glands located posterior to the thyroid, behind the upper pole of each thyroid lobe and at the level of or just below the lower pole of the thyroid. Variations, including ectopic locations are not uncommon.

13.059 The function of the parathyroid glands is to
A. secrete thyroid hormone:
B. concentrate and release calcium from the parathyroid glands
C. regulate calcium ion concentration in the interstitial fluid
D. all of the above
E. B and C only

C. is correct.
Parathyroid glands regulate the calcium ion concentration by the synthesis and release of parathyroid hormone (PTH) which will stimulate the release of calcium from the skeleton, the GI tract (by absorption), and retention of calcium by the kidneys in the presence of lower than normal interstitial calcium concentration.

13.060 The indication for parathyroid imaging is the clinical diagnosis of:
A. hypoparathyroidism
B. hyperparathyroidism
C. hyperthyroidism
D. all of above
E. A and B only

B. is correct.
Hyperparathyroidism is characterized by an increase in the synthesis and release of PTH, resulting in elevated calcium levels. Primary hyperparathyroidism is most often the result of parathyroid adenomas. Imaging is most useful in pre-surgical localization of ectopic parathyroid glands.

13.061 The dual isotope technique for parathyroid scintigraphy employs the use of:
A. 201 Tl thallous chloride
B. ^{99m}Tc pertechnetate
C. 67Ga citrate
D. 111In oxine
E. A and B only
F. B and C only
G. A and C only

E. is correct.
Both 201 Tl thallous chloride and ^{99m}Tc pertechnetate are distributed through normal thyroid tissue. However, the concentration of thallium is greater in parathyroid adenomas and may be evidenced as increased uptake either by visual examination of the images or using computer subtraction techniques to subtract the thyroid tissue out.

13.062 If using the dual isotope technique and only a dual peak system is available, the 201 Tl energies that should be used are:
A. 135 keV
B. 167 keV
C. 69-83 keV
D. 140 keV
E. A and C
F. A and D
G. B and C
H. B and D

G. is correct.
Imaging on the 201Tl window can be accomplished by imaging the 69-83 keV characteristic x-rays alone or with the 167 keV gamma rays (8% abundance). If 3 energy windows are available, the 135 keV gamma Rays (2% abundance) may be added.

13.063 The usual dose of 201 Tl chloride for parathyroid imaging is in the range of:
   A. 500 uCi - 1 mCi
   B. 2 - 3 mCi
   C. 4 - 5 mCi
   D. 5 - 10 mCi

B. is correct.
The usual dose of 201 Tl chloride is in the range of 2 -3 mCi; the dose for the ^{99m}Tc pertechnetate is in the range of 5 -10 mCi.

13.064 Patient preparation for parathyroid imaging should include:
   A. NPO for at least 4 hours
   B. emphasizing the importance of not moving until the completion of the examination
   C. pretreatment with perchlorate to reduce the dose to the thyroid
   D. no patient preparation is needed

B. is correct.
The patient should be made aware of the importance of not moving from the beginning of the first computer acquired pinhole image (with 201 Tl) to the end of the second pinhole image (with ^{99m}Tc pertechnetate); approximately 45 minutes.

13.065 A single isotope technique for parathyroid imaging uses:
   A. 131I mIBG
   B. ^{99m}Tc PTH
   C. ^{99m}Tc sestimibi
   D. 67 Ga citrate

C. is correct.
Sestimibi will be taken up by both thyroid and parathyroid tissue; delayed imaging demonstrates clearance from the normal tissue in the glands, and persistence of activity in the abnormal parathyroid tissue.

13.066 The radiopharmaceutical used in bone marrow imaging is:
   A. ^{99m}Tc sulfur colloid
   B. ^{99m}Tc MAA
   C. ^{99m}Tc DTPA
   D. ^{99m}Tc HDP

A. is correct.
This is the same radiopharmaceutical that is used for liver-spleen imaging. It is phagocytized by the reticuloendothelial cells that are present in the liver, spleen, and bone marrow. ^{99m}Tc micro-aggregated albumin or other ^{99m}Tc tracers that are picked up by the RES may be useful. (111In chloride).

13.067 The adult dose for bone marrow imaging is:
   A. 2-3 mCi
   B. 5 mCi
   C. 10-15 mCi
   D. 20 mCi

C. is correct.
The adult dose of 10 mCi (370 MBq) is increased over the usual 5 mCi liver spleen imaging dose to increase the relative dose to the bone marrow. (Approximately 75-80% of the dose goes to the liver).

13.068 In spot views of the thoracic and lumbar spine, it is usually a good idea to include as much of the liver in the view as possible.
   A. true
   B. false

B. is correct.
The lower thoracic and upper lumbar spine are usually not well visualized because of the high uptake of the liver and spleen; as little of the liver as possible should be included so that most of the counts are coming from the spinal bone marrow.

13.069 Indications for bone marrow scintigraphy may include all of the following EXCEPT:
   A. bone infarction
   B. avascular necrosis
   C. sickle cell anemia
   D. polycythemia
   E. osteoporosis

E. is correct.
Bone marrow imaging may be used to study the functional capacity of bone marrow and marrow space diseases. Osteoporosis is a reduction in the bone mass.

13.070 The dose to scan time for ^{99m}Tc sulfur colloid bone marrow imaging is:
  A. immediate
  B. 5 -10 minutes
  C. 60 minutes
  D. 2 hours
  E. 4-6 hours

C. is correct.
Waiting 1 hour before imaging will allow for maximum concentration of the radiopharmaceutical by the bone marrow. Some departments may choose to begin imaging earlier.

13.071 Hepatic artery catheters which deliver chemotherapeutic agents directly to the site of liver metastases can be evaluated for proper placement with the use of a:
  A. bolus intravenous injection of ^{99m}Tc pertechnetate
  B. bolus intravenous injection of ^{99m}Tc sulfur colloid
  C. slow injection of the chemotherapeutic agent into the infusion port
  D. slow injection of ^{99m}Tc MAA into the infusion port

D. is correct.
After administration of MAA, the drainage pattern of the hepatic catheter can be evaluated and ^{99m}Tc sulfur colloid can be injected intravenously to outline the liver and determine whether the placement of the catheter is perfusing the entire liver.

13.072 The imaging agent for adrenal cortical scintigraphy is:
  A. 131I hippuran
  B. 131I NP-59
  C. 131 (123) I mIBG
  D. all of above
  E. B and C

B. is correct.
131 (123)I NP-59 (6B iodomethylnorcholesterol) has been used to identify adrenomedullary disease. 131I NP-59 has a high affinity for the adrenal cortex.

13.073 Indications for imaging the adrenal cortex include all of the following EXCEPT:
  A. primary hyperaldosteronism
  B. adrenal hyperandrogenism
  C. pheochromocytoma
  D. adrenal lesions seen on CT, MRI, or US

C. is correct.
Pheochromocytomas are tumors, either benign or malignant of the adrenal medulla.

13.074 Patient preparation for adrenal cortical scintigraphy should include:
  A. NPO since midnight the night before
  B. pretreatment with Lugol's solution
  C. patient should be taken off tricylic antidepressants
  D. treatment with Lugol's throughout the study
  E. all of the above
  F. C and D only
  G. A, B, and D only

G. is correct.
Patients should be injected in a fasting state because of the possible interference of elevated serum cholesterol with the study. The Lugol's (or SSKI) is administered to prevent thyroid uptake of the 131I.

13.075 When imaging with 131I NP-59, if gallbladder activity is evidenced on the posterior view, the technologist should:
  A. take an anterior view
  B. take a lateral view
  C. have the patient take a drink of water
  D. take delayed images

B. is correct.
The lateral view with help to distinguish the gallbladder (an anterior structure) from the right adrenal.

13.076 The imaging agent for adrenal sympathomedulla scintigraphy is:
  A. 131I hippuran
  B. 131I NP-59
  C. (123) 131 I mIBG
  D. all of above
  E. B and C

13.077 Patient preparation should include:
  A. NPO from midnight on
  B. a bolus injection
  C. patient should be taken off oral contraceptives
  D. a careful medical history of medications

13.078 The appearance of the heart on a 131 I mIBG study is:
  A. a normal distribution
  B. evidenced only if levels of catecholamine are elevated
  C. an artifact
  D. due to improper radiopharmaceutical preparation

13.079 One of the potential risks or pitfalls associated with antibody imaging is:
  A. decreased sensitivity to detection
  B. tissue rejection
  C. anaphylaxis
  D. non-specificity

13.080 The indication for radionuclide venography is for the evaluation of:
  A. regional perfusion in organs and extremities
  B. deep venous thrombosis
  C. primary lymphedema
  D. all of the above
  E. B and C only

13.081 The usual route and technique of administration for radionuclide venography includes:
  A. simultaneous IV injection of 3 mCi of MAA into the dorsal vein of each foot
  B. simultaneous IV injection of 6 mCi of MAA into the dorsal vein of each foot
  C. injection of 1 mCi for each image (legs, thighs, and pelvis/lower abdomen), into the dorsal vein of each foot
  D. injection of 3 mCi for each image (legs, thighs, and pelvis/lower abdomen), into the dorsal vein of each foot

C. is correct.
131 I mIBG has been used to identify adrenomedullary disease and demonstrate the presence of pheochromocytoma and other catecholamine-secreting tumors. It has also proved useful in identification of tumors of neuroectodermal origin.

D. is correct.
Because of the large number of drugs that could interfere with or promote 131I mIBG uptake, patients should be off of medications for several weeks before imaging.

A. is correct.
The normal distribution of 131I mIBG includes the salivary glands, liver, spleen, and heart. Normal adrenal medulla is seldom visualized.

C. is correct.
A 1-mg dose of epinepherine should be available to treat anaphylaxis and the patient should be alerted to the potential allergic reactions and risks associated with the injection of a foreign protein. A detailed history of previous allergic reactions should be noted.

B. is correct.
The technique of radionuclide venography is to visualize the deep venous system of the lower extremity for the presence of deep venous thrombosis (DVT). While x-ray contrast venography is the "gold standard" for imaging the deep venous system, Doppler ultrasound is establishing its superiority and lacks the undesirable effects of the contrast venographic study.

C. is correct.
Usually both extremities are imaged simultaneously; the 6 mCi dose is contained in two syringes, one for each leg. Each 3 mCi dose should be in a volume of 3 ml so that 1 mCi can be injected for each image required.

13.082 Tourniquets may be applied at both the ankle and the knee for the purpose of:
    A. keeping the dose in the superficial venous system
    B. injecting into the iliac veins
    C. increasing the flow in the dorsum of the foot
    D. diverting the dose to the deep venous system

D. is correct.
The additional tourniquets are applied at the knees to divert the flow away from the superficial veins in the leg and into the deeper venous system.

13.083 An advantage to the alternative method of using of ^{99m}Tc tagged red blood cells to evaluate DVT, includes:
    A. arterial perfusion can be evaluated
    B. the injection can be in a vein in the arm
    C. fresh forming thrombi can be detected
    D. pulmonary emboli can be detected
    E. C and D
    F. A and B

F. is correct.
The area of interest can be evaluated for arterial perfusion aiding in the diagnosis of acute thrombophlebitis. The injection can be in the arm, avoiding the discomfort associated with a pedal injection. The deep as well as the superficial venous system can be evaluated with this technique.

SECTION 14: TUMOR AND INFECTION SCINTIGRAPHY

TUTORIAL

As defined by *Taber's Cyclopedic Medical Dictionary,* 16th edition, inflammation is tissue reaction to injury that may be the result of blows, foreign bodies, chemicals, electricity, heat or cold, microorganisms, surgery, or ionizing radiation. There are hemodynamic and permeability changes as well as a migration of leukocytes to the area of tissue damage. Infection is that state or condition of the body or part of the body that is invaded by a pathogen (microorganism or virus) that multiplies and produces injurious effects. Localized infection is usually accompanied by inflammation, but inflammation may occur without infection. A tumor is a spontaneous new growth of tissue forming an abnormal mass developing independent of, and unrestrained by normal laws of growth and morphogenesis.

In nuclear medicine, 67Ga citrate is used in imaging several tumors that are gallium avid such as lymphoma, hepatoma, seminoma, melanoma, and rhabdomyosarcoma. It has also been used in imaging for infection and abscess detection. It has been used in conjunction with conventional bone scanning in assessing and differentiating osteomyelitis from cellulitis. Gallium is also used to evaluate active inflammatory disease whether from infection or other etiologies.

111In leukocyte imaging takes advantage of the fact that leukocytes (white blood cells) accumulate in areas of infection. 111In labeled leukocytes are thought to be more sensitive than 67Ga citrate in acute infections. Since there is no bowel accumulation of 111In leukocytes, it is the radiopharmaceutical of choice for detection of abdominal infection. The patient's white cells are labeled, tagged with 111In and reinjected. Areas of accumulation outside the normal tracer activity (spleen, liver, and bone marrow) represent infection.

14.001 Gallium 67 has physical characteristics of:
  A. 4 day half-life
  B. decay by photoelectric effect
  C. 78 hour half-life
  D. decay by electron capture
  E. C and D

E. is correct.
67Ga has a 78 hour (3.25 day) half-life and decays by electron capture. In addition, it has four principal gamma ray energies.

14.002 Of the four principal radiation emissions of 67Ga, the greatest abundance is from the:
  A. 93 keV
  B. 184 keV
  C. 296 keV
  D. 393 keV

A. is correct.
40% of the gamma emissions arise from the 94 KeV energy; 24% from the 184 keV, 22% from the 296 keV, and 7% from the 393 keV.

14.003 The use of a medium energy collimator and a multiple window pulse height analyzer is necessary for gallium imaging in order to:
  A. reduce septal penetration of the higher energy peaks
  B. reduce scatter
  C. improve sensitivity
  D. all of the above

D. is correct.
Detection of multiple peaks will increase count sensitivity. At the higher energies, the medium energy collimator with thicker lead septa will reduce septal penetration and scatter.

14.004 Initial blood clearance of carrier-free 67Ga citrate is fairly rapid, on the order of _____ remaining in the blood at 3 hours post injection.
  A. 10%
  B. 15%
  C. 25%
  D. 50%

C. is correct.
67Ga binds to circulating serum proteins (transferrin) following IV injection.

14.005 The 9-15% excretion of 67Ga citrate through the gastrointestinal system may require:
  A. adequate bowel preparation
  B. repeated views over successive days
  C. tomographic imaging of the abdomen
  D. all of the above

D. is correct.
There is question over the usefulness of enemas in 67Ga imaging; irritation of the bowel can mimic inflammation and the mechanism of bowel wall uptake may make the use of cleansing enemas ineffective. Sequential imaging to observe the movement of activity or tomography are effective means of distinguishing bowel activity from a site of inflammation or tumor.

14.006 Screening for fever of unknown origin (FUO) is an indication for 67Ga citrate imaging.
  A. true
  B. false

A. is correct.
Because 67 Ga localizes in either infection or tumor sites, it is the radionuclide of choice for screening for fever of unknown origin, especially in chronic conditions.

14.007 When scanning for tumor or metastatic disease with 67Ga citrate imaging, one should take into account:
  A. the biologic half-life of the agent
  B. accumulation in recent biopsy or surgical sites
  C. renal accumulation
  D. cross-scatter in multi-window registration

B. is correct.
Recent biopsies or surgeries should be noted because 67Ga citrate may accumulate in biopsy or surgical sites.

14.008 In cases of infection, abscesses may be evident in 67Ga scintigraphy as soon as:
  A. 1-2 hours
  B. 4-6 hours
  C. 24-36 hours
  D. 48-72 hours

B. is correct.
Initial imaging in abscess detection should take place at 6 hours post injection.

14.009 In situations of lymphoma or lung inflammations, 67Ga imaging is most useful as:
  A. an initial diagnostic process
  B. a staging and follow-up of therapy
  C. an alternative to CT
  D. the sole diagnostic modality

B. is correct.
It is generally believed that the degree of lung uptake correlates with the degree of activity of the inflammation or tumor.

14.010 A combination of ^{99m}Tc and 67Ga imaging is a more desirable imaging technique than radiographs in cases of osteomyelitis.
  A. true
  B. false

A. is correct.
67Ga and 111In-labeled leukocytes are used in adjunct to ^{99m}Tc-phosphonate 3- or 4-phase bone imaging to increase the specificity in diagnosing osteomyelitis. A normal gallium image excludes osteomyelitis.

14.011 Gallium 67 scanning has found increased routine use in the evaluation of the following pulmonary conditions EXCEPT:
   A. sarcoiditis
   B. interstitial lung disease
   C. pneumococcal pneumonia
   D. metastatic breast CA
   E. Acquired immunodeficiency disease

D. is correct.
Localization of gallium in metastatic breast cancer has been inconsistent in tumor identification.

14.012 Planar 67Ga imaging of the chest includes which of the following pitfall(s)?
   A. over and underlying activity of sternum and spine
   B. lack of precise depth determination of active foci
   C. poor target to background ratios
   D. hilar activity versus mediastinal disease differentiation
   E. all of the above
   F. A and C only

E. is correct.
The use of SPECT imaging with 67Ga eliminates some of the pitfalls encountered with planar imaging.

14.013 The identification of the depth and extent of gallium-avid foci is easily visualized with the use of SPECT imaging.
   A. true
   B. false

A. is correct.
High-count imaging with multi-headed equipment will facilitate the identification and localization of lesions enhanced with gallium.

14.014 If a 67Ga scan and three-phase bone scan using ^{99m}Tc-phosphonate are ordered to rule-out osteomyelitis, what general protocol for injection and scanning should the technologist follow?
   A. inject the ^{99m}Tc-phosphonate, image flow, inject 67Ga, image ^{99m}Tc bone scan at 2-4 hours, image 67Ga at 6-24 hours
   B. inject 67Ga, inject the ^{99m}Tc-phosphonate, image flow, image ^{99m}Tc bone scan at 2-4 hours, image 67Ga at 6-24 hours
   C. inject 67Ga, image 67Ga at 6-24 hours, inject the ^{99m}Tc-phosphonate, image flow, image ^{99m}Tc bone scan at 2-4 hours
   D. inject the ^{99m}Tc-phosphonate, image flow, image ^{99m}Tc bone scan at 2-4 hours, inject 67Ga, image 67Ga at 6-24 hours

D. is correct.
Injecting 67Ga before the ^{99m}Tc-phosphonate study is accomplished will result in increased background from the gallium. The 67Ga should be injected after the bone scan images have been obtained.

14.015 The technologist observes renal activity on gallium images performed within 24 hours of IV injection of carrier free gallium. The most likely explanation for this activity is:
   A. infection or inflammation of the kidneys
   B. severe hepatocellular disease
   C. normal finding
   D. a misadministration of the dose
   E. all of the above

C. is correct.
Gallium uptake in the kidneys within 24 hours of administration demonstrates normal localization of the radionuclide.

14.016 Doses of 5 - 10 mCi of 67 Ga would be:
   A. within normal limits for imaging studies
   B. a misadministration
   C. used only if SPECT images are to be obtained
   D. used for tumor imaging only

A. is correct.
Dose limits of 5-10 mCi (185-370 MBq) are within range for most imaging departments.

14.017 Which of the following radionuclides has demonstrated higher sensitivity for chronic inflammatory lesions?
  A. 67Ga citrate
  B. 111In leukocytes
  C. ^{99m}Tc phosphonates
  D. ^{99m}Tc RBCs
  E. 201Tl

A. is correct.
While 111In leukocytes are more sensitive for acute inflammation, 67Ga has the higher sensitivity for chronic inflammatory lesions.

14.018 Which of the following organs does NOT concentrate 111In labeled leukocytes?
  A. bowel
  B. lung
  C. liver
  D. spleen

A. is correct.
One of the advantages of 111In in examining the abdomen is its lack of concentration in the gastrointestinal tract.

14.019 The typical dosage of 111In used for leukocyte imaging is:
  A. 100 uCi
  B. 500 uCi
  C. 1.5 mCi
  D. 2-5 mCi

B. is correct.
Indium 111 is an active metal with an abundance of gamma emissions in the optimum range for detectability.

14.020 At approximately 24 hours post administration, the greatest concentration of 111In leukocyte activity would be in the:
  A. spleen
  B. liver
  C. bone marrow
  D. blood pool
  E. A, B, and C

E. is correct.
After the first 4 hours, localization is highest (20-50%) in the spleen, the liver, and the bone marrow. This relative distribution does not change after the first 4 hours.

14.021 The estimated radiation dose from 111In leukocytes is highest for which of the following organs?
  A. liver
  B. spleen
  C. bone marrow
  D. lungs

B. is correct.
Dose distribution for 111In labeled white blood cells follows the distribution or amount of red blood cells present. The spleen has the highest concentration of red blood cells and therefore the highest rad/mCi of dose administered.

14.022 The administration of 111In labeled leukocytes should be accomplished by:
  A. rapid injection through a higher gauge needle
  B. slow injection through a lower gauge needle
  C. slow injection through a plastic tubing infusion line
  D. rapid injection using a glass syringe

B. is correct.
Slow injection through a lower gauge (larger bore) needle decreases the trauma to the blood cells during injection. Plastic tubing should be avoided, and blood products can react with glass.

14.023 Which of the following radionuclides has demonstrated higher sensitivity for acute inflammatory lesions?
  A. 67Ga citrate
  B. 111In leukocytes
  C. ^{99m}Tc phosphonates
  D. ^{99m}Tc RBCs
  E. 201Tl

B. is correct.
111In leukocytes are more sensitive for acute inflammatory lesions and for imaging in the region of the bowel.

14.024 What additional imaging technique might be employed when imaging the the upper abdomen for abscesses with 111In leukocytes?
   A. 67 Ga quantification
   B. ^{99m}Tc sulfur colloid subtraction
   C. single pass whole body scanning
   D. delayed static images (72-96 hours post injection) of 111In leukocytes

B. is correct.
Because of the high activity in the liver and spleen, ^{99m}Tc sulfur colloid subtraction may be an option for imaging the upper abdomen for abscess localization.

14.025 The purpose of adding hetastarch to the collected blood sample is to:
   A. prevent the clotting of the red blood cells
   B. prevent the disassociation of the 111In oxine with the leukocytes
   C. act as a preservative for the sample
   D. bind any indium not labeled to the leukocytes
   E. increase the settling rate of the red blood cells

E. is correct.
The purpose of hetastarch (synthetic plasma volume expander) in the labeling technique is to increase the settling rate of the red blood cells. (Some departments may use a methyl cellulose solution to more thoroughly separate the RBCs).

14.026 In a situation where the patient does not have sufficient white cells in the peripheral blood:
   A. donor granulocytes may be tagged
   B. the study cannot be accomplished
   C. an arterial blood sample may be withdrawn
   D. a larger bore needle may be used to prevent trauma

A. is correct.
A donor who has been properly typed by a blood bank may provide granulocytes to be tagged or labeled using the 111In oxine technique.

14.027 One disadvantage associated with 111In white cell scans is:
   A. imaging the whole body is an alternative
   B. indium images are low count increasing acquisition time
   C. its sensitivity in inflammatory bowel disease
   D. the scans may be positive when other imaging modalities are negative

B. is correct.
Acquisition times of 5-10 minutes are appropriate for the low count images. Older patients and children may need special attention and instruction on the importance of holding still during the acquisition.

14.028 Special attention to what quality control parameter is of utmost importance when labeling blood products?
   A. camera performance
   B. dose calibration and assay
   C. labeling all tubes, syringes, and laboratory equipment with the appropriate patient identification
   D. radiochemical purity testing of the radionuclides used

C. is correct.
Universal precautions, infection control, and implementation of proper patient care techniques, demand absolute accuracy in patient identification of all materials associated with a blood labeling technique.

14.029 Production of radiolabeled products specific to individual tumor antigens are called:
   A. tumor surface antigens
   B. T lymphocytes
   C. hybridomas
   D. monoclonal antibodies

D. is correct.
Monoclonal antibodies are produced by a plasma cell that are specific to antigens on the tumor cell surface.

14.030 Immunoscintigraphy may provide a distinct advantage over CT and ultrasound by:
   A. demonstrating a palpable mass
   B. early detection of cancer before a palpable mass
   C. confirming the diagnosis of cancer on a radiographic mass
   D. both A and C
   E. none of the above

B. is correct.
Immunoscintigraphy has the capability of provide early detection and diagnosis of cancer before a palpable or radiographic mass is assessed.

SECTION 15: HEMATOLOGY AND NON-IMAGING PROCEDURES

TUTORIAL

The blood that is circulating to and from the body cells within the vessels of the vascular system varies in color from bright red to dull brick red depending upon the amount of oxygen it is carrying. The circulatory system of the average adult contains about 5.5 liters of blood. If blood is collected with an anticoagulant, the whole blood will separate into a fluid (plasma) compartment and a cellular compartment. In a collection without an anticoagulant, a clot will form and the straw-colored fluid that is separated from the clot is known as serum.

Plasma proteins include albumin, globulin, and fibrinogen. Red blood cells or erythrocytes primarily transport hemoglobin which is an oxygen-carrying pigment. The average life span of red blood cells is between 100-120 days. Senescent red blood cells are primarily destroyed in the spleen. White blood cells or leukocytes are the primary effector cells against inflammation and tissue damage. The platelets play an important role in blood coagulation, hemostasis, and blood clot formation.

The hematocrit which is the volume of erythrocytes packed by centrifugation in a given volume of blood and is expressed as the percentage of the total volume of blood that consists of red blood cells. The hematocrit reading can be misleading in estimating blood volume or in the determination of the true number of red blood cells circulating in the body. For example, if a patient is dehydrated and has a decreased plasma volume, there will be a falsely elevated hematocrit. If the plasma volume is increased, the hematocrit will be falsely low. Direct measurement of the circulating red cell volume and plasma volume using radiotracers have proven to be extremely accurate in measuring the plasma and red cell volume. Since red cell volumes are contained in a closed system, the isotope dilution principle is used for total blood volume measurements: $V = \dfrac{Q}{C}$, where,

V is volume, Q is the dose administered in counts per minute, and C is the concentration of the dose after dilution (in the body) in counts per minute. The red blood cells are randomly labeled using 51 Cr (sodium chromate). The plasma compartment may be labeled using 125I human serum albumin or ^{99m}Tc-labeled human serum albumin, although the ^{99m}Tc labeled human serum albumin must be 98% bound at time of injection.

Red cell survival and splenic sequestration studies if carefully performed can give an accurate indication of the mean survival time of red cells in patients with hemolytic anemia. Since the splenic sequestration study is usually performed in conjunction with the red cell survival study, it is also possible to determine if the spleen is the site of red cell destruction.

The vitamin B_{12} absorption or Schilling test helps to determine whether a patient is able to absorb orally administered vitamin B_{12}. Untreated, vitamin B_{12} deficiencies can include abnormalities of the bone marrow, GI, and neurological systems and affects the maturation of all tissues in the body. Pernicious anemia is the classic vitamin B_{12} deficiency syndrome.

15.001 The primary function of the erythrocytes is:
A. clotting mechanism
B. combating infection
C. oxygen-carrying system
D. regulation of the acid-base balance in the blood
E. C and D

E. is correct.
Erythrocytes (or mature red blood cells) carry oxygen and carbon dioxide. They also play a role in the regulation of the acid-base balance in the blood and in the formation of bile pigments, which are derived from the decomposition products of hemoglobin.

15.002 A cell with the primary function of combating infection is:
A. erythrocytes
B. blood platelets
C. leukocytes

C. is correct.
Leukocytes (or white blood cells) act as scavengers, cleaning up damaged cells and destroying organisms.

15.003 The volume of packed red blood cells that is expressed as a percentage of the blood sample is called the:
A. RBC differential
B. hematocrit
C. hemolyzed RBCs
D. plasmacrit

B. is correct.
The hematocrit value represents the ratio of the cellular component to the total volume of a sample of blood.

15.004 The grayish cell layer called the buffy coat, just above the red blood cells consists of:
A. erythrocytes
B. platelets
C. white blood cells
D. plasma

C. is correct.
The buffy coat contains the white cells in the sample of blood.

15.005 When using microhematocrit tubes, the technologist should insure that the reading is of packed red cells by:
A. using a thin marker to note the separation
B. measure the tube against a control tube
C. subtracting the volume of white blood cells and platelets
D. using a magnifying glass to read the tube

D. is correct.
A hand held magnifying glass or the magnifier attached to the centrifuge should be used to read the hematocrit values.

15.006 If a hematocrit is run on a woman with a value below 32%, it would be a good idea to:
A. repeat the hematocrit
B. call the attending physician
C. ask the patient if she is on iron pills
D. wait two weeks and run the test again

A. is correct.
A repeat hematocrit is run on women if the value lies below 32% and on men if the value lies below 35%. Generally, hematocrits are run in duplicate to insure accuracy.

15.007 The degree of packing of the cellular elements of the blood is affected by all of the following factors EXCEPT:
A. patients weight
B. speed of centrifugation
C. time of centrifugation
D. inadequate mixing of the blood
E. presence of tissue fluid (from finger prick)

A. is correct.
The weight of the patient does not have a direct effect on the degree of packing of the cellular element of the blood.

15.008 If blood is allowed to settle without an anticoagulant added, the _____ will be separated from the
A. plasma; cells
B. serum; clot
C. plasma; serum
D. serum; hemoglobin

B. is correct.
Blood without an anticoagulant will settle into a fluid component (serum) and a clot (cells and proteins).

15.009 When anticoagulated blood is centrifuged, the layers from top to bottom in the tube are:
A. serum, platelets, white blood cells, red blood cells
B. serum, white blood cells, red blood cells, platelets
C. plasma, red blood cells, platelets, white blood cells
D. plasma, platelets, white blood cells, red blood cells
E. red blood cells, white blood cells, platelets, plasma

D. is correct.
An anticoagulant added to whole blood and centrifuged will result in a plasma component and a cellular component consisting of platelets, white blood cells, and red blood cells.

15.010 If a patient's hematocrit is 45% and his total blood volume is 4900 ml, what will the patient's plasma volume be?
A. 245 ml
B. 2205 ml
C. 2450 ml
D. 2695 ml
E. 2940 ml

D. is correct.
The hematocrit represents the packed cell volume; therefore the plasma crit would be 55% (100 - 45 = 55). 55% of 4900 = 2695.

15.011 After centrifugation of a blood specimen, the serum is a clear red. This color:
A. indicates the presence of lipids or fats in the specimen
B. indicates the presence of lysed RBCs in the specimen
C. indicates the presence of elevated levels of bile pigments in the specimen
D. is the normal color of serum

B. is correct.
Serum is usually straw colored. Hemolysis (or decomposition of red blood cells) will cause the serum to look red.

15.012 When drawing a blood sample, all of the following could cause a blood specimen to hemolyse EXCEPT:
A. forceful spraying of the blood through the needle
B. using a small bore needle
C. leaving the tourniquet on the patient while drawing the specimen
D. poor venipuncture technique causing excessive trauma to the blood vessel

C. is correct.
Leaving the tourniquet on the patient while withdrawing blood will not injure the cells.

15.013 What percentage of distilled water is there in a serum sample that has been diluted 1:50, serum : water?
A. 10%
B. 25%
C. 50%
D. 98%
E. 105%

D. is correct.
The ratio of 1:50 represents 1 divided by 50 = .02. The serum is 2% of the sample, the distilled water is 100-2 = 98%.

15.014 If precise volume measurement of less than 5 ml is needed, the laboratory glassware that would be most appropriate is a(n)
A. Erlenmeyer flask
B. laboratory beaker
C. manual or automatic pipet
D. volumetric flask
E. graduated cylinder

C. is correct.
A volumetric flask can provide accurate measurements to + or - 0.001%. However, for small volumes, or where an appropriately sized flask is unavailable, the manual or automatic pipet delivers a precise volume.

15.015 The automatic pipet should have a % error of
    A. less than 1%
    B. 2%
    C. 3-5%
    D. 5-10%

A. is correct.
An accurate pipet should have an error of less than 1%; the CV (coefficient of variation) for precision of the instrument, should be 3% or less.

15.016 The analytic balance is used to determine:
    A. mass weights of small quantities
    B. the accuracy of automated pipets
    C. volume measurements of flasks
    D. mass weights of lead syringe shields

A. is correct.
The analytic balance measures mass weights of small quantities of solid materials.

15.017 Refrigerated centrifuges should be routinely checked for which of the following?
    A. correct revolutions per minute (rpms)
    B. G forces
    C. daily temperature checks
    D. all of the above
    E. A and C only
    F. B and C only

D. is correct.
In addition to periodic checks for correct rpms and G forces, daily temperature readings should be taken and recorded.

15.018 If materials in the lab need to be kept at a constant 40 degree temperature, which of the following should NOT be used?
    A. water bath
    B. frost-free refrigerator
    C. dry ice cooler
    D. liquid nitrogen thermos
    E. all of the above

E. is correct.
For all of the above there is the problem of large temperature changes occurring. For all water baths, freezers, and refrigerators used in the lab, daily temperature records should be maintained.

15.019 The pH of human blood must be maintained between:
    A. 6.2 - 6.8
    B. 6.9 - 7.1
    C. 7.3 -7.5
    D. 7.6 - 7.8

C. is correct.
Buffering systems in the body maintain the blood pH between a narrow range of 7.3 - 7.5.

15.020 The element that is essential in the synthesis of hemoglobin is:
    A. bilirubin
    B. iron
    C. potassium
    D. chromium

B. is correct.
Hemoglobin is the iron-containing pigment of the red blood cells.

15.021 A patient with a low platelet count would have difficulty:
    A. forming a blood clot
    B. producing antibodies for immunity
    C. combating infection
    D. with autoimmunity

A. is correct.
Platelets play an important role in blood coagulation and thrombus formation after an injury.

15.022 If a patient is dehydrated, the effect on the hematocrit would be that:
    A. the hematocrit is falsely lowered
    B. the hematocrit is falsely elevated
    C. the hematocrit is unaffected by dehydration of the patient

B. is correct.
If a patient is dehydrated, the plasma volume will decrease and the ratio of plasma to red blood cells will reflect a falsely elevated packed cell count or hematocrit reading.

15.023 In a patient with a gastrointestinal bleeding site, one would expect which of the following changes in blood volumes?
- A. plasma volume will increase; red cell mass will decrease
- B. plasma volume will decrease; red cell mass will increase
- C. plasma volume will increase; red cell mass will increase
- D. plasma volume will decrease; red cell mass will decrease
- E. none of the above

A. is correct.
In bleeding, the blood volume decreases, cardiac output and arterial pressure decrease. The kidneys will retain fluid to bring the blood volume back within normal limits. These mechanisms increase the plasma volume to bring the total blood volume back to normal, but the red cell mass remains low.

15.024 Assume you have a radioactive sample with 65,000 cpm/ml. Take 1 ml of this sample and put it into an unknown volume of water. Mix and withdraw 1 ml and count. The number of counts is 1203 cpm/ml. Determine the volume of water in the unknown sample.
- A. 36 ml
- B. 43 ml
- C. 54 ml
- D. 78 ml
- E. 185 ml

C. is correct.
The relationship between concentration and volume is expressed as $C_1 \times V_1 = C_2 \times V_2$ or $V_2 = \dfrac{C_1 V_1}{C_2}$ so, $V_2 = \dfrac{65,000 \times 1\ ml}{1203} = 54$ ml.

15.025 Radionuclide tracers used in blood volume determinations nay either be tagged to the erythrocytes or to the:
- A. serum
- B. albumin
- C. platelets
- D. leukocytes

B. is correct.
Leukocytes and platelets are not easily measured in the cellular compartment. Radiolabeled albumin is used in the measurement of plasma volume.

15.026 Radiolabeling of red blood cells for red cell volume measurement is considered a:
- A. cohort label
- B. hematocrit label
- C. leukocyte label
- D. random label

D. is correct.
The labeling process involves labeling all erythrocytes circulating in the peripheral blood regardless of age. This "random" label tags the youngest to the oldest cells in the sample.

15.027 Falsely high results on a red blood cell volume may be found if:
- A. dose is extravasated
- B. the patient has had a previous administration of a radiotracer
- C. the sample is drawn from the same site as the injection of the dose
- D. the equipment is contaminated with radioactivity

A. is correct.
If the entire dose is not injected into the vein (part is extravascular), or the RBCs are damaged, the values received will be erroneously high. Falsely low values will be obtained as a result of B, C, or D.

15.028 The radiopharmaceutical of choice to label red blood cells for a study that is evaluating red cell volume is:
- A. ^{99m}Tc pertechnatate
- B. 51Cr sodium chromate
- C. 111In oxine
- D. 125I labeled serum albumin

B. is correct.
Although ^{99m}Tc pertechnatate has physical characteristics that make it nearly ideal for RBC volume determinations, the fact that it elutes rapidly from the RBCs does not make it a feasible alternative when studies must extend beyond a 60 minute sampling time. Therefore the radiopharmaceutical of choice is 57Cr sodium chromate.

15.029 The usual dose of 57Cr that is used for the measurement of circulating red blood cell mass is:
   A. 5 uCi
   B. 10 uCi
   C. 1 mCi
   D. 5 mCi

B. is correct.
Statistically valid sample counts can be obtained with a 10 uCi dose of 57Cr.

15.030 Ascorbic acid is added to the cell labeling vial for the purpose of:
   A. reducing the hexavalent chromate ion
   B. oxidizing the trivalent chromic ion
   C. reducing the free chromate to chromic ion
   D. tagging the platelets in the vial

C. is correct.
The reduction of free chromate to chromic ion in the tagging vial stops the tagging process as the chromic ion is unable to cross the red blood cell membrane.

15.031 If a patient has a disease state that may delay mixing of the tagged sample with the circulating blood, the most appropriate action would be to:
   A. withdraw a sample from the vein not used for injection, after 10 minutes
   B. withdraw a sample from the vein used for injection, after 10 minutes
   C. wait 24 hours before withdrawing the postinjection sample
   D. take serial samples until there is no significant difference in successive counts

D. is correct.
In seriously ill patients, patients with spenomegaly or severe polycythemia, delayed mixing may occur. Taking serial samples will insure that complete mixing has occurred before the postinjection sample is obtained.

15.032 The radiopharmaceutical that is used for the estimation of plasma volume is:
   A. ^{99m}Tc pertechnatate
   B. 51Cr sodium chromate
   C. 111In oxine
   D. 125I labeled serum albumin

D. is correct.
125I labeled human serum albumin tags the plasma potion of blood.

15.033 Multiple heparinized samples of blood are withdrawn at timed intervals in a plasma determination for the purpose of:
   A. reducing the error of random sampling
   B. extrapolating the physical decay of the 125 I
   C. reducing the radiation load in the patient
   D. establishing the rate of diffusion of the albumin from the vascular system

D. is correct.
The tagged albumin will diffuse into extravascular compartments in the same manner as untagged proteins.

15.034 Total blood volume and plasma volume measurements are limited by the fact that:
   A. normal values are difficult to predict accurately
   B. recent exercise and cold weather tend to decrease the plasma volume
   C. pregnancy and warm weather tend to increase the plasma volume
   D. obesity or recent weight loss affect the estimate from height and weight charts
   E. all of the above
   F. B and C only

E. is correct.
All of the factors listed are limitations of these studies. For this reason it is best to record the plasma volume as estimated.

15.035 In the erythrocyte survival and splenic sequestration studies, the radiopharmaceutical used is:
  A. ^{99m}Tc pertechnatate
  B. 51Cr sodium chromate
  C. 111In oxine
  D. 125I labeled serum albumin

B. is correct.
The red blood cells are labeled using 51Cr sodium chromate. The dose is adjusted by weight (generally not more than 1.5 uCi/kg of body weight).

15.036 The mean half-time of normal 51Cr-labeled RBCs is _____ days.
  A. 120
  B. 80 - 100
  C. 50 - 60
  D. 25 - 35
  E. 10 - 15

D. is correct.
The true mean half-time of senescent or aging cells is between 50 - 60 days (at a rate of 1% per day removal of the old cells from circulation). This is combined with a 1% per day elution of the 51 Cr label from the red blood cells which gives us a mean half-time of 25 - 35 days.

15.037 The primary indication for performing a red cell survival study is:
  A. polycythemia vera
  B. hemolytic anemia
  C. pernicious anemia
  D. leukocytopenia

B. is correct.
Hemolytic anemia results form the hemolysis of red blood cells. The survival study may be performed to determine the life span of red cells or to study the effect of therapy on patients with hemolytic anemia.

15.038 The red cell survival is often performed in conjunction with what other nuclear medicine study(s)?
  A. splenic sequestration
  B. red cell volume
  C. Vitamin B$_{12}$ absorption
  D. all of the above
  E. A and B only

E. is correct.
This study is often performed in conjunction with the red cell volume study and the splenic sequestration study since the red cells are labeled by use of the same technique.

15.039 Which day of the week should the nuclear medicine technologist try to schedule a red cell survival study?
  A. Monday
  B. Tuesday
  C. Thursday
  D. Friday

A. is correct.
Since samples are obtained every other day for three weeks, starting the examination on a Monday will allow for specimens to be obtained on Monday, Wednesday, and Friday of each week. (Also, the first sample is withdrawn 24 hours post injection - Tuesday).

15.040 The rate of production and destruction of RBCs can be affected by:
  A. increased or decreased fluid intake during the study
  B. acute blood loss during the time of the study
  C. blood transfusions administered during the time of the study
  D. all of the above
  E. B and C only

E. is correct.
Increased production of red blood cells, blood transfusions, or acute blood losses during the time of the study can give falsely decreased half-time results for the RBC survival time.

15.041 The reason for performing the splenic sequestration study in conjunction with the red cell survival study is to:
  A. evaluate the role of the spleen in decreased red cell survival
  B. determine occult blood loss
  C. indicate concurrent polycythemia vera
  D. all of the above

A. is correct.
A progressive increase in counts over the spleen indicates active sequestration of the 51Cr labeled red blood cells.

15.042 In active splenic sequestration of red blood cells, the ratio of spleen to liver counts may be:
   A. less than 1:1
   B. 2:1 or greater
   C. attributable to technologist error
   D. not determined with the available data

B. is correct.
Normally, the spleen to liver ratio is approximately 1:1; this rises to 2:1 or greater in patients with active splenic sequestration.

15.043 Patient preparation for a splenic sequestration examination should include having the technologist:
   A. explain that all counts will be taken in the prone position
   B. mark the patient's skin over the heart, liver, and spleen with indelible ink
   C. inform the patient that blood transfusions may be necessary
   D. all of the above

B. is correct.
To insure that counting geometry is maintained, the patient's skin should be marked with indelible ink and the probe placed on the exact same area of the body for each count.

15.044 The most appropriate collimator for use in counting in the splenic sequestration study would be the _____ collimator.
   A. pinhole
   B. high resolution
   C. flat field
   D. converging
   E. high sensitivity

C. is correct.
The flat field collimator limits the probe's field of view to a region of interest, providing uniform detection sensitivity and excluding most radioactivity outside of the region of interest so that the liver, spleen, and heart can be counted.

15.045 The splenic sequestration study will be invalid if:
   A. blood loss causes a shortened half-life
   B. blood transfusions are administered within the time of the study
   C. the probe is positioned inaccurately over the organs of interest
   D. all of the above
   E. A and C only

C. is correct.
Improper counting geometry may cause results to be spurious. Neither A nor B will affect the outcome of the splenic sequestration study.

15.046 Failure to absorb dietary B_{12} results in systemic symptoms related to:
   A. polycythemia vera
   B. pernicious anemia
   C. thrombosis
   D. leukemia

B. is correct.
Pernious anemia results from a deficiency in the gastric secretion of intrinsic factor, necessary for absorption of vitamin B_{12}.

15.047 The primary route of excretion for B_{12} that is not utilized by, or stored in the body, is through the:
   A. saliva
   B. bile and gallbladder
   C. urine
   D. feces
   E. pancreas

C. is correct.
The primary route of excretion is through the urine. If malabsorption occurs, the B_{12} may be excreted in the feces, rather than being absorbed in the terminal ileum and excreted in the urine.

15.048 The vitamin B_{12} absorption (Schilling Test) is performed as a(n) _____ test.
   A. in vivo
   B. in vitro
   C. radioimmunoassay
   D. antibody

A. is correct.
The vitamin B_{12} absorption test would be an in vivo test; the labeling is occurring in the body.

15.049 It is recommended that two separate 24 hour urine collections be obtained after the single flushing dose of B_{12} in instances where:
A. the patient may have urinary retention
B. the serum creatinine level is above 2.5 mg/dL
C. the first 24 hour collection may be incomplete
D. urinary function is not intact
E. all of the above
F. A and C only

E. is correct.
Significant amounts of radioactivity maybe excreted over 48 hours in patients with compromised urinary function. The second 24 hour collection will also help to verify if the first 24 hour collection was incomplete.

15.050 Patient preparation for the vitamin B_{12} absorption test should include clear instructions for the patient to include all of the following points EXCEPT:
A. overnight fasting
B. parenteral B_{12} should not be given for at least 3 days prior to the test
C. the importance of a complete 24 hour urine collection
D. the need for a hematocrit to test for radioactivity from previous medical tests
E. the fasting should be for 2 hours after the dose for the exam

D. is correct.
The hematocrit would not determine previous administration of radioactivity. It would be advised to have the patient empty his/her bladder before the test and obtain a patient urine sample at that time to test for radioactivity from previous exams.

15.051 The radioactive isotopes used currently to label vitamin B_{12} include _____ and _____ and are administered
A. 57Co & 60Co; intravenously
B. 57Co & 60Co; orally
C. 57Co & 58Co; intravenously
D. 57Co & 58Co; orally

D. is correct.
60Co was used in early studies, but currently 57Co and 58Co are preferred because of their shorter half-life and lower radiation dose. (57Co, 270 days, 122 keV; 58Co, 72 days, 810 keV)

15.052 The flushing dose of unlabeled B_{12} is administered:
A. intramuscularly
B. intravenously
C. intraperitoneally
D. intrathecally

A. is correct.
Two hours after the oral administration of .5uCi of 57Co vitamin B12, 1 mg of stable vitamin B12 is administer intramuscularly.

15.053 The purpose of the parenteral flushing dose of stable (non-labeled) B_{12} is to:
A. supplement the oral dose
B. to stimulate the secretion of intrinsic factor
C. to saturate the normal vitamin B12 binding sites in the circulating plasma
D. block fecal excretion of the labeled vitamin B12

C. is correct.
Unless this flushing dose is administered, there will be no activity found in the urine of normal or vitamin B_{12} deficient patients.

15.054 Vitamin B_{12} deficiencies may be due to:
A. failure of the stomach to secrete intrinsic factor
B. malabsorption syndrome
C. intestinal bacterial overgrowth, as in "blind loop" syndrome
D. parasitic competition
E. inadequate dietary intake
F. all of above
G. A and E only

F. is correct.

15.055 If the flushing dose of stable vitamin B_{12} were not administered, the results of the Shilling test would be:
   A. falsely high
   B. falsely low
   C. falsely normal
   D. unaffected

B. is correct.
The results would be falsely low as no activity would be counted in the urine. The excretion would be primarily through the feces.

15.056 Which of the following samples would contain the highest amount of labeled vitamin B_{12} if a Schilling test was performed on a vitamin B_{12} therapy patient?
   A. urine
   B. plasma
   C. feces
   D. packed RBC

C. is correct.
If large amounts of vitamin B_{12} are administered, it may be possible to block all the absorptive sites in the terminal ileum. A delay of 24-48 hours is usually a sufficient delay (before performing a Schilling test), in a patient with normal renal function.

15.057 Which of the following sources of error in the Schilling test will increase the percent excretion result?
   A. incomplete urine collection
   B. stable vitamin B12 not administered
   C. fecal contamination of the urine sample
   D. patient receiving vitamin B12 therapy

C. is correct.
We are looking to measure only that vitamin B_{12} that was absorbed in the terminal ileum and excreted through the urine.

15.058 What condition(s) might exist before a stage II Schillings test is administered?
   A. less than 6% 24-hour dose excretion
   B. 3 - 7 days must elapse
   C. greater than 9% 24-hour dose excretion
   D. both A and B

D. is correct.
An average of 5 days (3-7 days) should elapse before the test is repeated with intrinsic factor. A normal stage I test would have a 24-hour dose excretion of greater than 8-9%.

From the following Schilling test results, select the most likely condition responsible for the excretion results:

Percent Excretion

	Schilling Stage I	Schilling Stage II
Patient # 1	5%	4%
Patient # 2	6%	11%
Patient # 3	15%	14%
Patient # 4	8%	8%

15.059 Patient # 1; results would indicate:
   A. normal
   B. pernicious anemia
   C. intestinal malabsorption
   D. inconclusive results

C. is correct.
If the stage II represents a true abnormal result that rules out extrinsic factor dependent malabsorption, then other causes of malabsorption should be determined, treated, and followed by a repeat Schilling test.

15.060 Patient # 2; results would indicate:
   A. normal
   B. pernicious anemia
   C. intestinal malabsorption
   D. inconclusive results

B. is correct.
Patient # 2 had normal excretion results when treated with intrinsic factor, confirming the diagnosis of pernicious anemia.

15.061 Patient # 3; results would indicate:
   A. normal
   B. pernicious anemia
   C. intestinal malabsorption
   D. inconclusive results

A. is correct.
The excretion results on patient # 3 are above 8-9% indicating a normal Schilling test.

15.062 Patient # 4; results would indicate:
   A. normal
   B. pernicious anemia
   C. intestinal malabsorption
   D. inconclusive results

D. is correct.
The results on patient # 4 would be considered inconclusive or low normal.

SECTION 16: RADIONUCLIDE THERAPY

TUTORIAL

The nuclear medicine technologist is responsible for the implementation of proper radiation safety practices for all patients in the department including those patients being treated with radionuclides. Guidelines and regulations of the U.S. Nuclear Regulatory Commission should be conformed to as well as the use of the ALARA principles for employees and patients alike.

Receipt and storage of radionuclide therapy materials should be monitored and shielded. In the case of liquid 131I sources, the material should be stored in a fume hood because of the volatile nature of the material. All materials should be assayed at time of receipt.

Informing the patient of what will be happening during the administration of the dose, and in the case of a therapy dose greater than 30 mCi, the subsequent isolation, will gain the patients cooperation and compliance to the restrictions. Most patients would rather have several persons tell them what is going to happen, than have healthcare professionals assume that either the patient has been informed by their attending physician or someone else has told them what to expect.

All members of the hospital staff who will be in contact with a therapy patient should be aware of the specific concerns of the radionuclide they are dealing with. In the case of 131I therapy in excess of 30 mCi, if the patient is hospitalized, the private room will be posted with a "Caution: Radioactive Materials" sign that contains information as to the amount of time that nurses can attend the patient and that visitors are allowed to remain in the area.

Therapy with 32P colloid, has by virtue of its beta emissions, different radiation safety concerns. Nursing staff should be alerted to the possible contamination of bandages used at the site of therapy instillation and treat all dressings as if contaminated. The radiation safety officer (or chief nuclear medicine technologist, depending on the institution) should assume responsibility for notifying nursing staff and supervising the changing or removal of dressings used.

Title 10, Code of Federal Regulations of the Nuclear Regulatory Commission states that personnel dealing with therapy patients must receive radiation safety instruction concerning: visitor and patient control, waste management, contamination control, and notification of the radiation safety officer in case of emergency. All personnel should be familiar with the procedures for therapy patients in their department.

16.001 The greatest difficulty in calculating a physiologically appropriate therapeutic dose of radioiodine for thyroid disease is in determining the:
  A. percent thyroid uptake
  B. biological half-life
  C. effective half-life
  D. weight of the thyroid gland

D. is correct.
The weight of the thyroid gland is estimated based on physical exam and thyroid imaging.

16.002 Characteristics of an ideal therapeutic radiopharmaceutical include all of the following EXCEPT:
  A. significant or total beta emissions
  B. low energy particles
  C. moderately long half-life (days)
  D. minimal radiation dose to personnel and visitors

B. is correct.
Medium to high energy particles will effectively destroy cells in the target organ.

16.003 The degree of irradiation resulting from an internally located source of radiation depends on:
  A. the type and energy of the radiation emitted
  B. its physical half-life
  C. its biological half-life
  D. all of the above
  E. A and C only

D. is correct.
While in imaging an ideal radiopharmaceutical would be a pure gamma emitter, with a reasonably short biological and physical half-life, in therapy, the ideal radiopharmaceutical would be a beta emitter with a relatively long-half-life to exert the greatest biological effect.

16.004 131I therapy is used to treat which of the following thyroid disorders?
  A. hyperthyroidism
  B. thyroid carcinoma
  C. hypothyroidism
  D. thyroiditis
  E. all of the above
  F. both A and B

F. is correct.
The result of radiation of the follicular cells of the thyroid gland causes decreased cell division, eventual cell death, and loss of hormone production with the intent of allowing the gland to resume a homeostatic production of thyroid hormone.

16.005 Patients undergoing radionuclide therapy should be isolated if the dose administered is greater than _____ mCi.
  A. 10
  B. 30
  C. 50
  D. 100
  E. 150

B. is correct.
The patient may be released from isolation if a reading less than 5 mrem/hr at 1 meter is obtained or if the calculated residual activity is less than 30 mCi.

16.006 Generally, the effects of a fixed dose versus a fractionated radiation dose will be:
  A. milder with the fixed dose
  B. milder with the fractionated dose
  C. as long as the total dose received is equal, the effects will be the same

B. is correct.
A fractionated dose will allow undamaged cells to reestablish themselves before the next dose is received. This could also make the fractionated dose less effective in certain treatments and increase the incidence of relapse.

16.007 The incidence of radioiodine induced hypothyroidism is greatest _____ following therapy for Graves' disease.
  A. immediately
  B. 6 - 12 months
  C. 1 - 2 years
  D. 5 years

B. is correct.
Approximately 20% to 30% of Graves' disease patients treated with radioiodine become hypothyroid the first year following therapy. The rate is approximately 3% per year thereafter.

16.008 When using 131I for thyroid therapy, it is the _____ emissions which are responsible for the therapeutic effect.
  A. alpha
  B. beta
  C. gamma

B. is correct.
The beta emissions (Eb = 188 keV) range is approximately 2mm and most of the dose is delivered directly to the thyroid gland.

16.009 The radioactive materials precaution sheet which is attached to the chart of the radionuclide therapy patients shall list all of the following EXCEPT:
  A. the predicted date of discharge
  B. the exposure rate at 1 meter from the patient
  C. the radionuclide administered
  D. the administered dose activity

A. is correct.
The nuclear medicine technologist should not try to predict when the patient will be released from isolation. Individuals will excrete the radioiodine at differing amounts.

16.010 Which of the following from a 131I therapy patient would contain the greatest amount of radioiodine?
   A. saliva
   B. urine
   C. feces
   D. sweat

B. is correct.
The greatest amount of radioiodine will leave the body through the urine.

16.011 Urine and excreta from a patient who received a therapeutic dose of 131I in excess of 100 mCi should be:
   A. collected and stored until the radioactivity reaches background levels
   B. collected and stored until the radioactivity is less than 30 mCi
   C. released into the sanitary sewer system as excreted
   D. collected and transported to a burial site with other radioactive waste

C. is correct.
The patient should be instructed to flush the toilet several times after use to dilute the radioactivity.

16.012 If a reading of 0.8 mrem/hour is made in a room next to the therapy patient, the best action would be:
   A. discharge the therapy patient from isolation
   B. move the patient in the adjacent room to another location
   C. check the reading with a different survey instrument
   D. limit visitors to 1 hour/day/visitor

B. is correct.
The dose rate to nearby patients should be less than 0.6 mrem/hour to insure that their dose rate does not exceed 100 mrem in 7 consecutive days.

16.013 A survey meter measurement at the bedside of a recently treated radioiodine therapy patient indicates an intensity of 24 mrem/hour. What is the length of time that a visitor or nurse could remain at the point where the reading was taken?
   A. 2 minutes
   B. 4 minutes
   C. 5 minutes
   D. 7 minutes

C. is correct.
2 mrem/hour is the exposure limit for non-occupational individuals; so

$$\frac{24\ mrem}{60\ min} = \frac{2\ mrem}{X};\ X = \frac{2\ mrem\ (60\ min)}{24\ mrem};$$

$$X = 5\ minutes$$

16.014 In the above example, what would be the most practical solution to allow visitors to remain in the room a longer time?
   A. the patient could be moved to a larger room
   B. the visitor could stand at the doorway of the room
   C. the visitor could wear a lead apron
   D. if the visitor is 18, there are no restrictions as to the amount of time spent

B. is correct.
Exposure rates at the doorway would be measured and the time allowed at the doorway would be longer because of the inverse square law. (Increasing the distance from the source of radiation decreases the radiation dose rate).

16.015 A 10 uCi dose of 131I was administered for a thyroid uptake study. If the patient's gland weighed 30 grams and their 24 hour uptake was 29%, what was the concentration (uCi/gm), of the 131I deposited in the gland?
   A. 9.7 uCi/gm
   B. 8.7 uCi/gm
   C. .097 uCi/gm
   D. .087 uCi/gm

C. is correct.
10 uCi x .29 = 2.9 uCi (in the gland);
$$\frac{2.9\ uCi}{30\ gm} = .097\ \frac{uCi}{gm}$$

16.016 In the radionuclide therapy patient's room, exposure rates are measured at which of the following locations?
   A. the patient's bedside
   B. adjacent room
   C. the doorway
   D. all of the above
   E. B and C only

D. is correct.
In addition to the above mentioned, radiation fields at the foot of the bed and at the curtain line may also be recorded.

16.017 What can be done to determine when a radionuclide therapy patient may be released from isolation?
   A. dose rate measurements can be taken
   B. the volume of urine that is excreted can be measured
   C. calculations based on the physical half-life of the radionuclide can be used to estimate the residual activity
   D. the patient can be imaged in the nuclear medicine department

A. is correct.

$$\frac{\text{dose rate at administration}}{\text{mCi dose administered}} = \frac{\text{dose rate at time X}}{\text{mCi dose remaining at time X}}$$

16.018 If a patient receives 150 mCi (5550 MBq) of 131I and the initial dose rate at 3 m immediately following the administration is 200 mrem/hr, how many mCi remain in the patient after 24 hours if the dose rate at that time is 75 mrem/hr?
   A. 20 mCi
   B. 28 mCi
   C. 44.6 mCi
   D. 56.3 mCi

D. is correct.
Using the formula in the above question:
$$\frac{200 \text{ mrem/hr}}{150 \text{ mCi}} = \frac{75 \text{ mrem/hr}}{X}$$

$$X = \frac{(150 \text{ mCi})(75 \text{ mrem/hr})}{200 \text{ mrem}} = 56.3 \text{ mCi}$$

16.019 The use of 131I in treating Graves' disease is acceptable for all patients over 18 years of age.
   A. true
   B. false

B. is correct.
Women who are pregnant or lactating should not be treated with radioactive iodine.

16.020 Dose calculations of 131I for toxic nodular goiter are less accurate than for Graves disease because:
   A. it is difficult to estimate the size of the gland
   B. low functioning nodules may have little uptake of the 131I
   C. relapses are more frequent after treatment than with Graves' disease
   D. all of the above

D. is correct.
Because of the nodularity of the gland and likelihood of substernal extensions, it is difficult to estimate the size of the gland for dose calculations. The nodules that were hypofunctioning on thyroid scans may have little or no uptake, and the incidence of recurrence is much higher than for Graves' disease.

16.021 A radionuclide therapy drug used for palliation of bone pain from metastatic disease in patients with breast, lung, or prostate carcinoma is:
   A. ^{99m}Tc MDP
   B. 89Sr chloride
   C. 201Tl Thallous chloride
   D. 32P chromic phosphate

B. is correct.
Approximately 80% of patients receiving 89Sr chloride for palliation of bone pain have experienced pain relief.

16.022 The usual route of administration for 89Sr chloride is:
   A. intravenous
   B. intramuscular
   C. intraperitoneal
   D. intrathecal

A. is correct.
An intravenous injection of between 40 uCi/kg (1.48 MBq/kg) to 60 uCi/kg (2.22 MBq) is the route of administration.

16.023 Strontium-89 chloride is an effective treatment for relief of metastatic bone pain because
  A. it stays in the area of normal bone
  B. it decays by gamma emission
  C.there is significant uptake in the areas of osteoblastic activity in bone
  D. all of the above
  E. B and C only

C. is correct.
The uptake in the osteoblastic skeletal metastases remains in high concentration for up to several months following treatment. Strontium-89 decays by beta emission which because of the relatively short range in tissues (~ 8 mm), makes it an ideal therapy agent.

16.024 The biodistribution of 89Sr chloride is very similar to:
  A. 201 Tl chloride
  B. ^{99m}Tc MDP
  C. ^{99m}Tc GH
  D. 111In oxine

B. is correct.
Comparison scans of ^{99m}Tc MDP and 89Sr chloride show similar biodistribution patterns.

16.025 The radionuclide treatment for polycythemia vera includes:
  A. intravenous injection of 32P Chromic phosphate
  B. intracavitary injection of 32P Chromic phosphate
  C. intravenous injection of 32P Sodium phosphate
  D. intracavitary injection of 32P Sodium phosphate

C. is correct.
32P Sodium phosphate is injected intravenously.

16.026 It is important for the person drawing the dose of 32P sodium phosphate to confirm that:
  A. the colloid is in suspension
  B. the dose is a clear liquid
  C. the dose in a 50 cc syringe
  D. a higher gauge needle is used for injection

B. is correct.
While 32P sodium phosphate is a clear liquid and is injected intravenously, 32P chromic phosphate is a cloudy, bluish-green, colloid suspension and should never be injected intravenously.

16.027 The usual dose range for treatment of polycythemia vera with 32P sodium phosphate is:
  A. 500-1000 uCi
  B. 1 - 2 mCi
  C. 3 - 5 mCi
  D. 5 - 10 mCi

C. is correct.
Three to five mCi (111 - 185 MBq) are administered intravenously.

16.028 32P chromic phosphate is used as radionuclide therapy for the treatment of:
  A. malignant pleural effusions
  B. malignant peritoneal effusions
  C. metastatic bone disease
  D. all of the above
  E. A and B only

E. is correct.
32P chromic phosphate has had the highest rate of success in patients with malignant effusions secondary to ovarian cancer. It is used for effusions in the pleural, pericardial, and peritoneal cavities.

16.029 The usual route of administration for 32P chromic phosphate is:
  A. intravenous
  B. intramuscular
  C. intracavity
  D. intrathecal

C. is correct.
For peritoneal effusions, 15 mCi mixed with saline is the usual dose. Pleural effusions are usually treated with a lower dose of approximately 10 mCi.

16.030 To insure that the radiocolloid therapy agent (32P chromic phosphate) will disperse and cover the wall of the cavity, _____ may be injected into the cavity first and imaged.
   A. 67 Ga citrate
   B. 201 Tl chloride
   C. ^{99m}Tc MDP
   D. ^{99m}Tc sulfur colloid

D. is correct.
A radiopaque contrast material can also be injected and a KUB taken, but the sulfur colloid technique can be accomplished just before the administration of the therapeutic radionuclide in the nuclear medicine department.

16.031 Good radiation safety measures when handling 32P would include:
   A. use of lead syringe shields
   B. use of lead containers to transport the dose
   C. both A and B
   D. neither A nor B

D. is correct.
Because of the high density of lead, using lead to shied the dose would increase the occurrence of the high energy Bremssrahlung radiation. The low penetrating power of 32P, which makes it ideal for therapy, also makes it easy to shield with plastic.

SECTION 17: FILM PROCESSING/QUALITY CONTROL

TUTORIAL

Film processing refers to the entire procedure of chemically processing the film in order to convert the latent image to a visible and permanent image. The processing cycle consists of developing, fixing, washing, and drying. Efficient operation of a nuclear medicine department includes the central location and quality control of the dark room and film processor.

Trouble-shooting the cause of films that have decreased gray scale, artifacts, or look chemically "off", is part of the technologist's responsibility in the evaluation of each film that is taken on a patient study. This is true for the matrix camera systems as well as laser cameras.

Automatic film processing systems consist of 3 basic components; a transport mechanism, a system of developing and fixing chemistry, and the film itself.

Film consists of film base and emulsion, the photosensitive layer. The base may be clear or tinted blue, which is thought to enhance contrast in the developed scintigraph. The base consists of silver bromide crystals suspended in gelatin which dissolves in hot water, but not in cold. The base may be coated on one side (single-emulsion film) or both sides (double emulsion film). Nuclear medicine film is single-sided emulsion and may be either clear or blue depending on the reading physician's preference.

Film is sensitive to heat, light, ionizing radiation, chemical fumes, pressure, rolling, bending, etc. and any one of these factors can cause an adverse effect on the film. Film is packed in metal foil to protect it from light and moisture. Storage of film should be on its side in a cool, dry place. High temperatures can cause a loss of contrast and produce fog. It is also important to use film with shorter expiration dates first, as film aging causes a loss in speed and contrast and can result in a mottled appearance on the developed film. Film should be withdrawn slowly from the carton or film cassette to avoid discharging static electricity. The three classifications of static commonly found on films are tree static, crown static, and smudge static. Tree static results from rapid motions building up a charge that is discharged when the film is touched. Crown static is most often the result of rapidly withdrawing a sheet of film from a new box of film, and smudge static occurs when a discharge follows a path that is started by dust or lint on the film.

The greatest aid in preventing static buildup is adding moisture to the air, although grounding the loading bench provides a simple solution to the problem in most cases.

17.001 The emulsion on medical sheet film consists of:
   A. silver nitrate and cellulose
   B. silver bromide and gelatin
   C. silver nitrate and gelatin
   D. cellulose and acetate

C. is correct.
Silver nitrate crystals are evenly distributed throughout the gelatin. Ionization causes "clumping" of the Ag^+ nitrate which results in the blackening of the film.

17.002 The type of film that is most often used for recording images (analog or digital) in a nuclear medicine department is:
   A. single emulsion film
   B. double emulsion film
   C. triple emulsion film
   D. all of the above are used

A. is correct.
Single emulsion film is used since only one side of the film is being exposed to light.

17.003 The notch felt on the upper right, or lower left corner on medical imaging film indicates:
   A. the edge of the film to be handled during cassette loading
   B. the emulsion side is facing you
   C. the emulsion side is away from you
   D. the type of film being used

B. is correct.
The notch is easily felt in the dark room and indicates the emulsion side is facing you.

17.004 Sheet film comes packed in a metal foil wrapper which helps protect the film from:
   A. moisture
   B. light
   C. heat
   D. A and B only
   E. B and C only

D. is correct.
The metal foil wrapper helps to keep out moisture and light.

17.005 Film images have diminished contrast (loss of gray scale) and a slight "pink" cast to the film base. What is the most likely cause of this problem?
   A. weak developer chemistry; low developer temperature
   B. weak developer chemistry; high developer temperature
   C. improper intensity settings
   D. low count rate

A. is correct.
If the input temperature is too low, or the developer chemistry is improperly mixed, images may demonstrate decreased contrast and be too light.

17.006 The purpose of the fixing solution is to:
   A. activate the developer
   B. stop the developing process
   C. add citric acid to the fixer
   D. preserve the integrity of the film base
   E. increase the intensity of the image development

B. is correct.
The purpose of the fixing solution is to stop the developing process, dissolve unexposed, undeveloped silver bromide, and to make the latent image permanent.

17.007 The most likely cause of a crescent-shaped artifact on film would be:
   A. over exposure of the image
   B. fogging due to lightleaks
   C. bending of the film during cassette loading
   D. excessive heat
   E. static

C. is correct.
Bending of the film will cause a crescent shaped artifact that corresponds to the mechanical damage of the emulsion.

17.008 The timer/delay at the beginning of the development process in an automated developer is to:
   A. prevent light leaks
   B. maintain a constant temperature
   C. prevent chemicals in the developer and fixer from mixing
   D. prevent films from sticking together

D. is correct.
The leading sheet of film can be overtaken by the following sheet causing a jam to occur if the timer/delay is ignored.

17.009 Processing chemicals should be constantly maintained (replenished) for all of the following reasons EXCEPT:

A. under replenishment can contribute to film transport problem in the processor
B. films can be too light with diminished contrast
C. films will be more susceptible to static
D. films can look "milky"

C. is correct.
Over or under replenishment can adversely affect the physical characteristics of the film and contribute to film jams. Incorrect replenishment of the developer can result in films that are too light and have diminished contrast and under replenishment of the fixer results in milky films since the fixer cannot sufficiently remove all of the silver bromide crystals. Static is most often due to low humidity.

17.010 The technologist notices that a series of films are fogged or darkened. What should be checked as a possible cause?

A. cracks in the filter on the safe light
B. date of film expiration
C. light leaks in the darkroom
D. contaminated developer
E. all of the above
F. A, B, and C only

E. is correct.
All of the above can cause films that are fogged or darkened.

17.011 For quality control purposes, which of the following should be checked regularly?

A. optical density
B. chemistry (solutions) replenishment rates
C. temperature controls
D. all of above
E. A and C only

D. is correct.
A regular schedule to check chemical change, temperature monitoring, and film or optical density should be maintained. In addition, preventive maintenance and processor cleaning schedules should be established.

17.012 When placing film in storage, the technologist should note the expiration date to insure that:

A. the foil wrap is moisture proof
B. the film was kept in a cool, dry environment
C. film with shorter expiration dates are used first
D. film with longer expiration dates are used first
E. film has an infinitely stable shelf-life and no expiration date is necessary

C. is correct.
Film should be used before the expiration date since aging film causes loss in speed and contrast; therefore film with a shorter expiration date should be placed in front and used first.

17.013 In filming the images, either analog or digital display, it is important for the technologist to insure that:

A. all structures of interest are on the gray scale
B. intensity is adjusted throughout the study to adjust for decreased counts
C. background is subtracted
D. all of the above

A. is correct.
It is important that all structures of interest are between black and white (on the gray scale). The other points may be more appropriate to acquisition or digital display only.

17.014 Film contrast is a property that refers to the:

A. overall blackness of the image
B. differences between the blacks and whites (gray scale)
C. ability to separate two points that lie next to each other
D. amount of distortion of the object being imaged
E. clearness or sharpness of the image

B. is correct.
Film contrast should reflect the gray scale; that is, images of low count density should be the lightest gray while high count structures would be the darkest gray.

17.015 Film that is used beyond the expiration date may result in a finished image that looks:
  A. mottled in appearance
  B. like a film exposed to static electricity
  C. pink in appearance
  D. none of the above

A. is correct.
Films may look mottled in appearance with a loss of contrast.

17.016 The quantity of silver ions which congregate at the point of ionization depends on:
  A. whether the film is single or double sided
  B. the degree of exposure received by the crystal of silver bromide
  C. the temperature of the developer
  D. the base composition of the film

B. is correct.
When a silver bromide crystal is struck by ionizing radiation or light, the crystal undergoes ionization into a silver ion. The silver ions migrate toward the area of the development and congregate there depending upon the degree of radiation exposure received.

17.017 All of the following are concerns when storing film EXCEPT:
  A. date of purchase and expiration date
  B. protection from ionizing radiation
  C. temperature and humidity of storage area
  D. manufacturer's lot number

D. is correct.
The manufacturer's lot number may be useful in tracking a problem with a shipment of film but is not essential information in storing of the film.

17.018 If a technologist consistently runs 14 x 17 inch films so that the replenisher microswitch is activated by 17 inches of film travel instead of 14 inches, the most likely result is:
  A. the films will jam
  B. the films will be overexposed
  C. there will be significant over replenishment
  D. an increase in the developer temperature

C. is correct.
Improper film feeding results in an over replenishment and a wasteful increase in the amount of solution used.

17.019 A technologist develops the first film before the rest of the study is completed and notes that the images are too dark. What is the best action for the technologist to take?
  A. adjust the intensity on subsequent images, but note the change on the films
  B. leave the intensity set as for the first image so all images can be compared
  C. repeat the study 24 hours later using the appropriate intensity settings
  D. reinject the patient immediately and restart the procedure

A. is correct.
The intensity should be kept constant throughout the study so that images can be directly compared. However, if the first film is found to be too light or too dark, the intensity should be adjusted and the change in intensity clearly indicated on the film for the reading physician.

17.020 The technologist performing a lung scan notices a circular artifact on the persistence scope during the anterior image acquisition. An appropriate action for the technologist to take would be:
  A. mark the location of the artifact on the image
  B. note the artifact beside the image and retake with the artifact removed, if possible
  C. perform obliques or lateral views if the artifact is an implant to document
  D. all of the above
  E. B and C only

E. is correct.
No marks should be made directly on the images, but a notation to the side of the image indicating an artifact is appropriate. If the artifact is the result of an external attenuator (e.g. pajama snaps, medallion, coins, etc.), remove and retake the image. If the attenuator is internal, (e.g. pacemakers, implants), obliques and laterals will help to resolve the image.

17.021 If a patient is unable to hold still or is to be imaged in a position that is different that departmental procedure dictates, the technologist should:
   A. check with the nuclear medicine physician before proceeding with the study
   B. have the patient sedated for the study
   C. indicate on the patient's requisition and films any specific conditions that affected the images
   D. cancel the study and reschedule the patient

C. is correct.
The best action is to evaluate the patient and indicate on the film what specific conditions affected the acquisition of images. This will assist the physician who is initially interpreting the study and also be clear weeks or months later if the case is reviewed.

SECTION 18: MOCK EXAMINATION

18.001 Proper technique in administering a radiopharmaceutical includes:
  A. use of syringe shields
  B. use of disposable gloves
  C. recapping syringe needles that have been in contact with patients
  D. all of above
  E. A and B only

18.002 The radiopharmaceutical of choice to label red blood cells for a study that is evaluating red cell volume is:
  A. ^{99m}Tc pertechnatate
  B. 51Cr sodium chromate
  C. 111In oxine
  D. 125I labeled serum albumin

18.003 A 20 mCi dose of ^{99m}Tc HDP results in a total body absorbed dose of approximately 0.25 rads. This value is equivalent to:
  A. 0.25 rem
  B. 2.50 mGy
  C. 0.50 mSv
  D. 0.25 Gy

18.004 Which of the following is the reason most frequently cited on a bone scan requisition?
  A. location and extent of primary bone tumor
  B. location and assessment of extent of metastatic bone lesions
  C. determination of the extent of arthritic disease
  D. evaluate osteomalacia

18.005 P-32 has a half-life of 14.3 days. A sample has an original activity of 200 mCi. How much will be left after 3 days? (decay factor = .8644)
  A. 173 mCi
  B. 175 mCi
  C. 179 mCi
  D. 184 mCi

18.006 What is the danger in imaging patients in the standing position?
  A. one cannot get the camera close to the patient's surface
  B. the patient may become hypotensive and fall
  C. the camera does not operate properly and images will demonstrate asymmetry
  D. the patient may contaminate the collimator

18.007 Patient motion is one of the most common artifacts on SPECT studies. The most effective way for the technologist to detect motion is to:
  A. use a filter
  B. evaluate the raw planar images in cine format
  C. ask the patient if they moved
  D. subtract a larger area of background

18.008 The purpose of administering "cold" (unlabeled) PYP for red blood cell labeling with ^{99m}Tc is:
  A. to utilize the reducing agent in the pyrophosphate kit
  B. to cool the red blood cells to obtain maximum labeling efficiency
  C. to prevent clotting of the blood during the labeling process
  D. to increase the length of time that the label remains intact to allow for multiple views

18.009 A uniform response to a wide range of radioactivities is a parameter of dose calibrator performance known as:
  A. accuracy
  B. precision
  C. linearity
  D. geometric calibration

18.010 Which of the following protocols would maximize the counts coming from the testicles?
  A. place a lead shield over the thighs, prop testes on a towel over the shield, position camera anteriorly, inject bolus ^{99m}TcO4-, image
  B. tape penis up on abdomen, place a lead shield over the thighs, prop testes on a towel over the shield, position camera anteriorly, inject bolus ^{99m}TcO4-, image
  C. tape penis up on abdomen, prop testes on a towel over the shield, position camera anteriorly, inject bolus ^{99m}TcO4-, image
  D. position camera under the testes, inject bolus ^{99m}TcO4-, image

18.011 If a technologist is unsure about performing a study that is ordered on a patient's requisition, the technologist should:
  A. confirm the study with the patient
  B. confirm the study with the floor nurse
  C. obtain clarification from the requesting physician
  D. obtain clarification from the nuclear medicine physician
  E. C or D
  F. none of the above

18.012 The nuclear medicine technologist notices the appearance of esophagus and stomach on a DTPA aerosol ventilation scan. The most appropriate response is to:
A. prepare a new kit of DTPA and re-administer to the patient
B. check the particle size of the aerosol
C. continue the scan; this is a typical finding
D. change the tubing and check the nebulizer for cracks
E. have the patient hold their breath during re-administration of the dose

18.013 If you work in an area where a major part of your body could receive greater than 5 mrem in any one hour or more than 100 mrem in five consecutive days, the sign posted would be:
A. Caution: Radiation Materials
B. Caution: Radiation Area
C. Caution: High Radiation Area
D. no signage is necessary

18.014 Errors in measurement of the thyroid gland made when using a pinhole collimator may occur due to:
A. long acquisition time
B. small matrix size
C. incorrect orientation
D. parallax error
E. all of the above

18.015 Energy resolution of a NaI detecting system increases with increasing gamma ray energy. Expressed as %FWHM, this means that the %FWHM _____ as gamma energy increases.
A. increases
B. decreases
C. remains the same

18.016 When performing hepatobiliary imaging, the best view to separate the gallbladder activity from activity in the duodenum is the:
A. left anterior oblique
B. right anterior oblique
C. left lateral
D. right lateral
E. posterior

18.017 When a technologist is setting up for a SPECT acquisition, selection of the acquisition time should include consideration of:
A. the computer memory available
B. the speed of the processing program
C. the patient's ability to hold still
D. the resolution required for the study
E. A and C only
F. C and D only

18.018 Some considerations for possible errors that could contribute to an undiagnostic SPECT CNS brain scan include:
A. patient comfort and immobility for the duration of the study
B. patient to detector distance
C. environmental stimuli during the injection
D. artifacts from poor quality control technical factors
E. all of the above

18.019 Materials that should be considered potentially infectious for the organisms that transmit hepatitis B or AIDS include all of the following EXCEPT:
A. gauze caked with dried blood from an arterial puncture procedure
B. urine dipsticks
C. used phlebotomy needles
D. fluids from a suction canister in the intensive care unit
E. blood-soaked paper towels used in cleaning up a spill

18.020 Patient preparation for adrenal cortical scintigraphy should include:
A. NPO since midnight the night before
B. pretreatment with Lugol's solution
C. patient should be taken off tricylic antidepressants
D. treatment with Lugol's throughout the study
E. all of the above
F. C and D only
G. A, B, and D only

18.021 When testing MAA and using acetone as an ITLC solvent, free ^{99m}Tc is evident at the:
A. solvent front
B. relative front
C. origin
D. centerpoint

18.022 Records established on April 1, 1996, on ^{99}Mo breakthrough tests on elutions from the ^{99}Mo/^{99m}Tc generator elutions must be kept for a period of _____ year(s), or until April, _____.
A. one; 1997
B. two; 1998
C. three; 1999
D. four; 2000
E. five; 2001

18.023 What additional imaging technique might be employed when imaging the the upper abdomen for abscesses with 111In leukocytes?
   A. 67 Ga quantification
   B. ^{99m}Tc sulfur colloid subtraction
   C. single pass whole body scanning
   D. delayed static images (72-96 hours post injection) of 111In leukocytes

18.024 It is important for the person drawing the dose of 32P sodium phosphate to confirm that:
   A. the colloid is in suspension
   B. the dose is a clear liquid
   C. the dose in in a 50 cc syringe
   D. a higher gauge needle is used for injection

18.025 If a patient is unable to hold still or is to be imaged in a position that is different that departmental procedure dictates, the technologist should:
   A. check with the nuclear medicine physician before proceeding with the study
   B. have the patient sedated for the study
   C. indicate on the patient's requisition and films any specific conditions that affected the images
   D. cancel the study and reschedule the patient

18.026 A vial contains ^{99m}Tc at a concentration of 58 mCi / ml. A dose of 15 mCi is desired. How many ml should be withdrawn into the syringe? (i.e., What volume is required?)
   A. 0.26 ml
   B. 2.6 ml
   C. 0.39 ml
   D. 3.9 ml
   E. 0.87 ml

18.027 In the ^{99m}Tc polyphosphate bone image, the inferior tips of the scapulae can easily be mistaken for:
   A. rib lesions
   B. xipoid lesion
   C. metastatic lung tumor
   D. breast lesions

18.028 What is the easiest and most practical way for a technologist to reduce the radiation exposure from patients injected for nuclear medicine studies?
   A. lead shielding and lead aprons
   B. distance
   C. limitation of time of exposure
   D. concrete shielding

18.029 The radionuclide treatment for polycythemia vera includes:
   A. intravenous injection of 32P Chromic phosphate
   B. intracavitary injection of 32P Chromic phosphate
   C. intravenous injection of 32P Sodium phosphate
   D. intracavitary injection of 32P Sodium phosphate

18.030 Total blood volume and plasma volume measurements are limited by the fact that:
   A. normal values are difficult to predict accurately
   B. recent exercise and cold weather tend to decrease the plasma volume
   C. pregnancy and warm weather tend to increase the plasma volume
   D. obesity or recent weight loss affect the estimate from height and weight charts
   E. all of the above
   F. B and C only

18.031 Persistent pulmonary activity and poor visualization of the left side of the heart represent _____ during a first pass evaluation.
   A. a ventricular aneurysm
   B. a left - to- right intracardiac shunt
   C. a right - to - left intracardiac shunt
   D. pulmonary hypertension

18.032 Patients with obstructive pulmonary disease may show an aerosol scan appearance:
   A. that mimics the appearance of pulmonary emboli
   B. that results in central airway deposition of the radiopharmaceutical
   C. that results in a false negative study
   D. all of the above

18.033 Patient preparation for renal scanning includes:
   A. NPO after midnight
   B. well- hydrated
   C. NPO 4 hours prior to injection
   D. no preparation is necessary

18.034 If an area of increased activity is demonstrated on a whole body 131I metastatic survey in the area of the lower pelvis or upper thigh, the technologist should:
   A. consult the nuclear medicine physician for further views
   B. have the patient remove clothing from that area and wash the skin
   C. have the patient return for delayed views
   D. have the patient drink several glasses of water

18.035 Factors which delay the appearance of the gallbladder during hepatobiliary imaging are:
A. impairment of hepatocyte function
B. obstruction of the cystic duct
C. contraction of the gallbladder due to recent food ingestion
D. obstruction of the biliary ducts proximal to the cystic duct
E. all of the above
F. B and D only

18.036 In the radionuclide ventriculogram, the word image matrix which provides the best compromise between image resolution and memory required to store images is:
A. 64 x 64
B. 128 x 128
C. 256 x 256
D. none of the above

18.037 General principles of environmental asepsis apply to all of the following EXCEPT:
A. always clean from the least contaminated area toward the more contaminated area
B. always clean from the top down
C. avoid raising dust
D. always clean from the more contaminated area toward the least contaminated area

18.038 Reoxidation of ^{99m}Tc may be reduced by packaging the nonradioactive reagent kit in:
A. an oxygen atmosphere
B. a nitrogen atmosphere
C. a hydrogen atmosphere
D. a moisture-free atmosphere

18.039 A radiopharmaceutical kit is prepared at 11:00 AM with 3 ml of ^{99m}Tc pertechnatate from generate eluate that is calibrated for 600 mCi / 5 ml at 6:00 AM. How much activity will the kit contain? (The 5 hour decay factor is 0.561)
A. 1011 mCi
B. 360 mCi
C. 202 mCi
D. 120 mCi
E. 67 mCi

18.040 When performing a brain scan using ^{99m}Tc pertechnatate, a technologist notes that the patient had a previous bone scan within 24 hours. What might be the result of the current brain scan?
A. may be a false positive
B. may be a false negative
C. the choroid plexus will show
D. the increase background will make the scan unreadable

18.041 If the mean particle size of the radiocolloid prepared for liver and spleen scintigraphy is reduced:
A. spleen uptake is reduced
B. spleen uptake is increased
C. bone marrow uptake is reduced
D. bone marrow uptake is increased
E. both A and D
F. uptake is not affected by particle size

18.042 A patient's salivary glands may be stimulated with each of the following EXCEPT:
A. gum
B. lemon juice
C. water
D. perchlorate

18.043 At approximately 24 hours post administration, the greatest concentration of 111In leukocyte activity would be in the:
A. spleen
B. liver
C. bone marrow
D. blood pool
E. A, B, and C

18.044 Which of the following sources of error in the Schilling test will increase the percent excretion result?
A. incomplete urine collection
B. stable vitamin B_{12} not administered
C. fecal contamination of the urine sample
D. patient receiving vitamin B_{12} therapy

18.045 Factors that should be considered by the technologist in an effort to apply the ALARA principle to patients include:
A. administration of the correct dose of radiopharmaceutical to the patient
B. proper calibration of the dose calibrator to ensure its accurate performance
C. appropriate quality assurance tests on imaging equipment to ensure proper function
D. all of the above
E. both A and B

18.046 When performing quality control tests of constancy, accuracy, linearity, and geometric variation, the NRC directs correction by repair, replacement, or use of correction factors, if the error is greater than:
A. 5%
B. 10%
C. 15 %
D. 20%

18.047 If a shoulder or hip appears to have increased uptake not relevant to the the patient's history or complaint, the technologists first concern should be to:
  A. alert the attending physician to the problem
  B. ask the patient to roll on their side
  C. take oblique images of the affected area
  D. insure that the patient is lying flat and that the camera head is not angled

18.048 The in-vivo labeling technique for gated blood pool imaging is preferred in some institutions due to:
  A. its increased labeling efficiency
  B. its increased technical difficulty
  C. its greater target to non-target ratio
  D. all of the above
  E. none of the above

18.049 On radionuclide imaging, testicular torsion is often demonstrated by:
  A. decreased flow; photopenic area on delayed imaging
  B. increased flow; photopenic area on delayed imaging
  C. increased flow; hyperperfused area on delayed images
  D. decreased flow; hyperperfused area on delayed images

18.050 Drawbacks to 133Xe ventilation imaging include all of the following EXCEPT:
  A. low gamma photon energy (80 keV)
  B. a trap or exhaust is needed to remove the gas
  C. all phases of ventilation can be assessed
  D. patient cooperation is essential

18.051 Occasionally, a thyroid nodule will appear "hot" or "normal" on a ^{99m}Tc pertechnatate scan and "cold" on an iodine scan. This may be best explained by the fact that:
  A. the nodule did not organify the iodine
  B. the nodule did not trap the pertechnatate
  C. the nodule organified the iodine
  D. The nodule trapped the iodine

18.052 If only three views can be obtained during spleen imaging the best views to obtain are:
  A. anterior, left and right laterals
  B. posterior, left and right laterals
  C. anterior, posterior, and right lateral
  D. anterior, posterior, and left lateral

18.053 When preparing to scan a patient to be injected with a perfusion SPECT radiopharmaceutical, it is a good idea to:
  A. leave the room lights on to keep the patient alert
  B. dim the lights and let the patient relax
  C. immobilize the patient's head
  D. position the camera far enough from the patient's head so that the camera will not frighten him/her
  E. A, C, and D
  F. B and C only

18.054 The single isotope technique for parathyroid imaging uses:
  A. 131I mIBG
  B. ^{99m}Tc PTH
  C. ^{99m}Tc sestimibi
  D. 67 Ga citrate

18.055 In a situation where the patient does not have sufficient white cells in the peripheral blood:
  A. donor granulocytes may be tagged
  B. the study cannot be accomplished
  C. an arterial blood sample may be withdrawn
  D. a larger bore needle may be used to prevent trauma

18.056 What condition(s) might exist before a stage II Schillings test is administered?
  A. less than 6% 24- hour dose excretion
  B. 3 - 7 days must elapse
  C. greater than 9% 24-hour dose excretion
  D. both A and B

18.057 Strontium-89 chloride is an effective treatment for relief of metastatic bone pain because:
  A. it stays in the area of normal bone
  B. it decays by gamma emission
  C. there is significant uptake in the areas of osteoblastic activity in bone
  D. all of the above
  E. B and C only

18.058 Film that is used beyond the expiration date may result in a finished image that looks:
  A. mottled in appearance
  B. like a film exposed to static electricity
  C. pink in appearance
  D. none of the above

18.059 The ^{99}Mo column, if separated from a ^{99}Mo/^{99m}Tc generator, must be held for at least _____ prior to disposal as nonradioactive waste.
  A. 60.2 hours
  B. 10 days
  C. 660 hours
  D. 30 days

18.060 Of the following choices, which collimator is used for thyroid uptake studies with radio iodine?
A. flat field
B. diverging
C. converging
D. pinhole
E. medium energy

18.061 Which of the following considerations is NOT required for gastric emptying studies acquired and processed by computer?
A. premedication with antacids
B. correction for radioactive decay
C. geometric correction for depth and position of stomach
D. patient motion correction
E. B and C

18.062 When a physician orders "NPO" for a patient, this means that:
A. all urine samples must be saved
B. only water and ice chips are to given by mouth
C. intravenous therapy is to be given
D. nothing is to be given by mouth
E. the patient may walk to the bathroom

18.063 Which of the following may cause malabsorption of vitamin B_{12}?
1 antibiotics
2 steroids
3 excessive alcohol consumption
A. 1 and 2
B. 1 and 3
C. 2 and 3
D. 1, 2, and 3

18.064 ^{99m}Tc sulfur colloid localizes in functional liver tissue as a result of:
A. active transport
B. phagocytosis
C. capillary blockade
D. cell sequestration

18.065 A vial contains 260 mCi in 20 ml of fluid. How many ml should be withdrawn to obtain 20 mCi?
A. 0.07
B. 0.65
C. 1.30
D. 1.54
E. none of the above

18.066 A 57Co capsule is dissolved in 50 ml of water. How many ml should be withdrawn to make a 10% standard?
A. 2.5
B. 5.0
C. 10.0
D. 25.0

18.067 The organ receiving the greatest radiation dose using ^{99m}Tc phosphate bone imaging agent is:
A. bones
B. kidneys
C. bone marrow
D. bladder
E. liver

18.068 The QRS complex represents the:
A. depolarization of the ventricles
B. repolarization of the ventricles
C. the resting state of the ventricles
D. the beginning of the SA-node stimulation

18.069 The best way for a technologist to decontaminate a ^{99m}Tc pertechnatate spill to the hands is by the use of:
A. decay
B. alcohol
C. soap and water
D. an alkaline cleanser

18.070 The resolving power of collimators decreases with increasing gamma ray energy because of:
A. increased Compton scatter
B. increased geometric losses
C. increased septal penetration
D. decreased stopping power

18.071 Normalization of nuclear medicine images allows for:
A. the amount of data acquisition time to be shortened
B. simultaneous acquisitions in the posterior and anterior positions
C. simultaneous acquisitions and processing
D. comparison of information from different size regions of interest

18.072 The technologist performing a lung scan notices a circular artifact on the persistence scope during the anterior image acquisition. An appropriate action for the technologist to take would be:
A. mark the location of the artifact on the image
B. note the artifact beside the image and retake with the artifact removed, if possible
C. perform obliques or lateral views if the artifact is an implant to document
D. all of the above
E. B and C only

18.073 If the patient continues to bleed once the needle is removed:
A. order a type and cross match
B. reapply the tourniquet
C. apply pressure to the site with a gauze pad until bleeding stops
D. gently massage the arm from wrist to elbow

18.074 A pediatric dose must be prepared for a patient undergoing a bone scan. It has been determined that the patient should receive 67% of the standard adult dose of 20 mCi. What is the dose in mCi that the patient should receive?
    A. 6.7 mCi
    B. 9.25 mCi
    C. 13.4 mCi
    D. 18.0 mCi

18.075 On April 4, a radiopharmaceutical is received and calibrated at 150 uCi/ml. What is the concentration in uCi/ml, on April 20? (T1/2 = 8 days)
    A. 150
    B. 75
    C. 50
    D. 37.5
    E. 18.75

18.076 Obtaining a patient history prior to bone scanning is relevant for all of the following EXCEPT:
    A. previous history of trauma
    B. previous radiation or chemotherapy
    C. medications the patient is currently taking
    D. location of pain patient is experiencing
    E. A and D only
    F. all can be relevant considerations

18.077 When assaying a patient dose, if the sample is elevated slightly in the dose calibrator, the dose read-out will be _____ .
    A. higher than the actual dose
    B. lower than the actual dose
    C. the same as the actual dose

18.078 Pixel size is determined by:
    A. zoom factor
    B. time per image
    C. number of images acquired
    D. matrix size
    E. A and D
    F. B and D

18.079 The technologist notices that a series of films are fogged or darkened. What should be checked as a possible cause?
    A. cracks in the filter on the safe light
    B. date of film expiration
    C. light leaks in the darkroom
    D. contaminated developer
    E. all of the above
    F. A, B, and C only

18.080 A 10 mCi source of 201 Tl thallous chloride in a volume of 5 ml, calibrated for June 10, at 12 noon EST, was received on June 9. What would be the activity on June 9, at 1:00 PM EST? (pre-calibration decay factor for 25 hours = 1.26)
    A. 1.6 mCi/ml
    B. 2.52 mCi/ml
    C. 7.9 mCi/ml
    D. 12.6 mCi/ml

18.081 The biodistribution of 89Sr chloride is very similar to:
    A. 201 Tl chloride
    B. ^{99m}Tc MDP
    C. ^{99m}Tc GH
    D. 111In oxine

18.082 The purpose of the parenteral flushing dose of stable (non-labeled) B_{12} is to:
    A. supplement the oral dose
    B. to stimulate the secretion of intrinsic factor
    C. to saturate the normal vitamin B_{12} binding sites in the circulating plasma
    D. block fecal excretion of the labeled vitamin B_{12}

18.083 Venting of 133Xe gas to the atmosphere is acceptable in all of the conditions EXCEPT:
    A. a rooftop designated as a restricted area
    B. an activated charcoal filter is used as a trap
    C. the activity released is 10% or less of legal requirements
    D. all of above

18.084 A package arrives with a half-life of 8 days and a total quantity of 30 mCi. According to the NRC regulations:
    A. a wipe test is necessary
    B. the package is exempt from wipe test requirements
    C. the NRC should be notified immediately
    D. the package should be returned to the carrier

18.085 If the radioactivity of a ^{99m}Tc sample is 40 mCi at 8:00 AM, what will the activity of the sample be at 8:00 PM?
    A. 80 mCi
    B. 20 mCi
    C. 15 mCi
    D. 10 mC

18.086 A bone scan is performed on a patient with metastatic colon cancer. The scan demonstrates focal soft tissue activity in the right upper quadrant. The most likely explanation for this activity is:
    A. soft tissue inflammation
    B. female breast activity
    C. liver metastases
    D. myocardial infarction

18.087 A major disadvantage of ^{99m}Tc-PYP imaging is:
- A. the radiation dose to the patient
- B. the insensitivity of the test to distinguish between infarct and ischemia
- C. patient cardiac motion
- D. the delay between imaging and onset of symptoms

18.088 A dose equivalent of 20 mSv is equal to:
- A. 1 mrem
- B. 2 mrem
- C. 1 rem
- D. 2 rem

18.089 A 10 mCi dose of a radionuclide would be equal to what activity in becquerels?
- A. 3.7 Bq
- B. 37 Bq
- C. 370 Bq
- D. 37 MBq
- E. 370 MBq

18.090 In addition to spatial resolution, what other parameter of the detection system can be assessed with either a bar or orthogonal hole phantom?
- A. sensitivity
- B. uniformity
- C. spatial linearity
- D. geometric variation

18.091 Which of the following is not necessary for an ERPF (effective renal plasma flow) calculation?
- A. pre and post injection syringe counts
- B. patient's height
- C. patient's weight
- D. renal ROI counts
- E. all are needed

18.092 210uCi of 131 I hippuran is to be used on May 3. There was 300 uCi on the date of the assay, April 29. Is the activity present on May 3 acceptable for the prescribed dose? (decay factor = 0.651)
- A. no, because the activity remaining is less than 50% of the prescribed dose
- B. yes, because the activity remaining is greater than the prescribed dose
- C. yes, because the activity remaining is within 10 % of the prescribed dose
- D. as long as a diagnostic study can be obtained, the dose is irrelevant
- E. none of the above

18.093 In a normal patient lying flat, the pulmonary blood flow is:
- A. more abundant in the base of the lung
- B. more abundant in the apex of the lung
- C. uniformly distributed throughout the lung, greater toward the posterior
- D. the patient's position does not influence the pulmonary blood distribution

18.094 The intensity of radiation is 100 mrem/hr at a distance of 9 feet from the source. The intensity at 3 feet from the source is _____ mrem/hour.
- A. 33.3
- B. 300
- C. 333
- D. 900

18.095 Exophthalmos is characteristic of which condition(s)?
- A. Grave's disease
- B. thyrotoxicosis
- C. hyperthyroidism
- D. all of the above
- E. A and C only

18.096 The most accurate and cost effective study to distinguish nonobstructive versus obstructive jaundice is seen in:
- A. magnetic resonance imaging (MRI)
- B. sonography
- C. ^{99m}Tc IDA imaging
- D. computed tomography (CT)
- E. B and D

18.097 Aluminum breakthrough in ^{99}Mo / ^{99m}Tc generators can be a problem because the aluminum ions can:
- A. cause the eluent to be nonsterile
- B. cause a low grade fever in patients who receive radiopharmaceuticals prepared with the 99mTc eluate
- C. affect the biodistribution and tagging reactions
- D. deliver an unnecessarily high dose to patients receiving preparations with the ^{99m}Tc eluate

18.098 Which of the following radiopharmaceuticals is NOT based on detecting a compromised blood-brain barrier?
- A. ^{99m}Tc pertechnatate
- B. ^{99m}Tc DTPA
- C. ^{99m}Tc GH
- D. 201 Tl
- E. ^{99m}Tc HMPAO

18.099　An area of expanded blood pool is noted on a GI bleeding scan using ^{99m}Tc labeled RBCs. It is located in the center of the abdomen and maintains its relationship to the aorta on an LAO view. This activity is most likely due to:

A. an active bleed
B. aortic aneurysm
C. inflammatory bowel disease
D. small bowel bleeding

18.100　An ultrasound examination demonstrates an incidental liver mass. The patient is referred for a 3-phase liver scan using ^{99m}Tc labeled RBCs. The results reveal an area of hypoperfusion and increased delayed blood pool images. This pattern is indicative of:

A. hepatoma
B. cyst
C. cavernous hemangioma
D. metastases

18.101　When using microhematocrit tubes, the technologist should insure that the reading is of packed red cells by:

A. using a thin marker to note the separation
B. measure the tube against a control tube
C. subtracting the volume of white blood cells and platelets
D. using a magnifying glass to read the tube

18.102　Patients undergoing radionuclide therapy should be isolated if the dose administered is greater than _____ mCi.

A. 10
B. 30
C. 50
D. 100
E. 150

18.103　In filming the images, either analog or digital display, it is important for the technologist to insure that:

A. all structures of interest are on the gray scale
B. intensity is adjusted throughout the study to adjust for decreased counts
C. background is subtracted
D. all of the above

18.104　What can be done to determine when a radionuclide therapy patient may be released from isolation?

A. dose rate measurements can be taken
B. the volume of urine that is excreted can be measured
C. calculations based on the physical half-life of the radionuclide can be used to estimate the residual activity
D. the patient can be imaged in the nuclear medicine department

18.105　Which of the following central nervous system studies is routinely used for the determination of brain death?

A. a blood brain barrier study using ^{99m}Tc DTPA
B. a cisternogram using 111In DTPA
C. a cerebral arteriogram using ^{99m}Tc MAA
D. all are routinely used

18.106　A patient injected with ^{99m}Tc MDP and scanned 2 hours post injection demonstrated activity in the liver. This was most likely due to:

A. scanning too soon after injection of MDP
B. extravasation of the dose
C. presence of ^{99m}Tc-tin colloids
D. presence of free or unbound ^{99m}Tc pertechnatate

18.107　If a reversible defect is seen in the antero-septal and septal walls during 201Tl scintigraphy, it is most likely due to:

A. an occluded left circumflex artery
B. a narrowed left anterior descending artery
C. a narrowed right coronary artery
D. an occluded left anterior descending artery

18.108　Following the administration of a radiopharmaceutical for a diagnostic imaging study, the patient develops a high fever and chills. This is most likely a _____ reaction.

A. radiation
B. bronchogenic
C. pyrogenic
D. cardiovascular
E. anaphylactic

18.109　If a patient receives 150 mCi (5550 MBq) of 131I and the initial dose rate at 3 m immediately following the administration is 200 mrem/hr, how many mCi remain in the patient after 24 hours if the dose rate at that time is 75 mrem/hr?

A. 20 mCi
B. 28 mCi
C. 44.6 mCi
D. 56.3 mCi

18.110　The dose for a radionuclide gated blood pool study in your facility is 20 mCi of ^{99m}Tc pertechnatate. A patient is given a dose of 5 mCi of ^{99m}Tc pertechntate intravenously and a diagnostic study performed. The dose was:

A. a misadministration, the dose was more than 50% different from the prescribed dose
B. incorrectly administered by intravenous injection
C. correctly administered, as long as a diagnostic study is achieved
D. A and B

18.111 Of the choices given, the best dynamic acquisition parameters for a three-phase bone scan following the bolus intravenous injection of ^{99m}Tc MDP are:

A. 10 serial images of 1 minute each
B. 20 serial images of 3 seconds each
C. 30 serial images of 1 second each
D. 30 serial images of 60 seconds each

18.112 The nuclear medicine technologist discovers that the patient injected for a biliary scan has had an opioid drug administered for pain previous to coming to the department for the scan. What might be the expected result?

A. delayed visualization of the gallbladder
B. delayed visualization of the small bowel
C. delayed clearance from the common bile duct
D. all of the above
E. B and C
F. none of the above

18.113 When interpreting a lymphoscintogram, the evaluation is based on which of the following criteria?

A. the continuity of the lymphatic chain
B. the width of the radioactive chain
C. the intensity of the uptake
D. the topographic distribution of the radioactivity
E. the radioactivity within the liver
F. all of the above
G. A and C only

18.114 The filter algorithm selected by the technologist should include consideration of:

A. the preference of the interpreting physician
B. the target-to-nontarget ratio
C. the background or "noise" level
D. all of the above

18.115 The timer/delay at the beginning of the development process in an automated developer is to:

A. prevent light leaks
B. maintain a constant temperature
C. prevent chemicals in the developer and fixer from mixing
D. prevent films from sticking together

18.116 The paradoxical functional image of a RVG is best identified as:

A. arterial contraction
B. aneurysmal ventricular motion
C. hypokinetic areas of the myocardium
D. all of the above

18.117 180 mCi in 10 ml is added to 100 ml. The resulting concentration is:

A. 0.16 mCi /ml
B. 0.18 mCi /ml
C. 1.6 mCi / ml
D. 1.8 mCi /ml
E. 18 mCi / ml

18.118 While performing a venipuncture, transfixation can result in:

A. formation of a deep hematoma
B. syncope
C. hemoconcentration
D. nausea and vomiting

18.119 In order to count the 320 keV peak of Cr-51 with a 15% window the window should be set at _____ keV.

A. 15
B. 24
C. 30
D. 48

18.120 Although manufacturers may differ on uniformity correction flood techniques, the one recommendation by all vendors is:

A. use of a large, 57Co flood source
B. monthly acquisition of a correction flood
C. use of a high count flood correction matrix
D. use of refillable flood sources for 67Ga, 111In, and 123I

18.121 The quantity of silver ions which congregate at the point of ionization depends on:

A. whether the film is single or double sided
B. the degree of exposure received by the crystal of silver bromide
C. the temperature of the developer
D. the base composition of the film

18.122 Radioactive materials that decayed through ten physical half-lives are reduced to:

A. background
B. less than 5 mrem/hr
C. less than 2 mrem/hr
D. less than .2mrem/hr

18.123 In some nuclear medicine departments, _____ may be given to reduce the dose to the thyroid from ^{99m}Tc pertechnatate injected for testicular imaging.

A. potassium permanganate
B. potassium perchlorate
C. potassium sulfide
D. none of the above

18.124 What needs to be considered when injecting a dose of ^{99m}Tc MAA through plastic tubing or syringes?

A. the proportion of dose that never reaches the patient

B. mixing of the dose with patient blood

C. speed of injection

D. position of the patient

E. all of the above

18.125 Radiotracers used for evaluating the spleen include all of the following EXCEPT:

A. 111In labeled WBCs

B. ^{99m}Tc labeled RBCs, denatured

C. 111In oxine platelets

D. ^{99m}Tc sulfur colloid

E. 201 Tl chloride

F. ^{99m}Tc albumin colloid

18.126 A bone agent was prepared at 7:30 AM and a patient dose administered at 1:00 PM. The patient was scanned 2 hours post injection and the bone scan shows activity in the salivary glands and stomach. This activity is most likely due to:

A. scanning too soon after injection of MDP

B. extravasation of the dose

C. presence of ^{99m}Tc-tin colloids

D. presence of free or unbound ^{99m}Tc pertechnatate

18.127 The usual average dose for ^{99m}Tc-labeled SPECT perfusion imaging agents such as HMPAO (Ceretec) and ECD (Neurolite) is:

A. 3-5 mCi (111 -185 MBq)

B. 5-10 mCi (185-370 MBq)

C. 15 mCi (555MBq)

D. 20 mCi (740 MBq)

18.128 If the intensity of radiation is 10 mrem/hour at 2 meters from the source, the intensity at 8 meters from the source is _____ mrem/hour.

A. 0.625

B. 2.5

C. 40

D. 160

18.129 Which radiopharmaceutical listed below would be the best choice for determination of ventricular shunt patency?

A. 111 In DTPA

B. ^{99m}Tc DTPA

C. ^{99m}Tc MAA

D. ^{99m}Tc pertechnatate

18.130 Special attention to what quality control parameter is of utmost importance when labeling blood products?

A. camera performance

B. dose calibration and assay

C. labeling all tubes, syringes, and laboratory equipment with the appropriate patient identification

D. radiochemical purity testing of the radionuclides used

18.131 Percent energy resolution is defined or calculated as follows:

A. photo peak energy (keV) / FWHM (keV)

B. photo peak energy (keV) / FWHM (keV) X 100

C. FWHM (keV) / photo peak energy (keV)

D. FWHM (keV) / photo peak energy (keV) X 100

18.132 In general, the number of images acquired in a 360 degree SPECT acquisition is related to the size of the organ being imaged and the resolution of the imaging system.

A. true

B. false

18.133 A survey meter measurement at the bedside of a recently treated radioiodine therapy patient indicates an intensity of 24 mrem/hour. What is the length of time that a visitor or nurse could remain at the point where the reading was taken?

A. 2 minutes

B. 4 minutes

C. 5 minutes

D. 7 minutes

18.134 In the above example, what would be the most practical solution to allow visitors to remain in the room a longer time?

A. the patient could be moved to a larger room

B. the visitor could stand at the doorway of the room

C. the visitor could wear a lead apron

D. if the visitor is 18, there are no restrictions as to the amount of time spent

18.135 The most likely cause of a crescent-shaped artifact on film would be:

A. over exposure of the image

B. fogging due to lightleaks

C. bending of the film during cassette loading

D. excessive heat

E. static

18.136 Of the following, which will suppress thyroid uptake for the longest period of time?

A. synthroid

B. cough medications

C. IVP contrast

D. oral cholecystographic agents

18.137 The usual route of administration of ^{99m}Tc pertechnatate for joint imaging is:
   A. intravenous
   B. intramuscular
   C. intrathecal
   D. intraperitoneal

18.138 Upon arrival, a package containing radioactive material with a DOT Category II yellow label must have a dose rate which at the surface does not exceed:
   A. .5 mrem/hour
   B. 5 mrem/hour
   C. 25 mrem/hour
   D. 50 mrem/hour

18.139 Accurate assessment of cardiac ejection fractions can be obtained with a minimum of:
   A. 8 frames
   B. 16 frames
   C. 20 frames
   D. 32 frames

18.140 Patients who suffer from orthopnea need to have:
   A. padding under bony prominences
   B. their heads elevated in order to breathe
   C. the feet elevated to avoid pain
   D. restraints applied to avoid falls
   E. a skin graft

18.141 A vial contains 350 mCi of ^{99m}Tc in 30 ml of fluid. What is the concentration?
   A. 11.7 mCi / ml
   B. 1.17 mCi / ml
   C. 0.86 mCi / ml
   D. 0.09 mCi / ml

18.142 The remaining ^{99m}Tc that remains untagged after the preparation of ^{99m}Tc MDP are:
   A. radionuclidic impurities
   B. radiochemical imuriities
   C. colloidal impurities
   D. pyrogenic impurities
   E. chemical impurities

18.143 Which of the following statements is NOT true regarding the labeling of 111In oxine white blood cells (WBC)?
   A. all traces of plasma should be removed before labeling.
   B. the In+3 will pass through the WBC membrane
   C. the 111In-labeling technique requires aseptic technique.
   D. it is necessary to withdraw 30 to 50 ml of blood from the patient.

18.144 The following occurs as filtered air is introduced into the ^{99m}Tc MAG3 reaction vial during the boiling phase:
   A. pH is stabilized
   B. reduction of the Mertiatide compound
   C. progressive formation of labeled impurities
   D. oxidation of excess stannous ions

18.145 For a 15% window (photo peak 320), the baseline of the SCA should be set at:
   A. 296
   B. 305
   C. 320
   D. 368

18.146 Personnel radiation exposure records should be kept:
   A. indefinitely
   B. 2 years
   C. 3 years
   D. 5 years

18.147 The mechanism of localization of ^{99m}Tc PYP in the necrosed myocardial tissue is best explained by:
   A. the deposition of potassium in the damaged myocardial cell
   B. the deposition of calcium in the damaged myocardium
   C. mitochondrial accumulation of denatured proteins
   D. all of the above
   E none of the above

18.148 In a gated cardiac scan, the patient's heart rate is 60 beats per minute. If each cardiac cycle is divided into 20 equal time segments , the average time will be ____milliseconds long.
   A. .05
   B. 0.5
   C. 5.0
   D. 50

18.149 Two radiopharmaceuticals that can be used to measure the effective renal plasma flow (ERPF) include 131I hippuran (OIH) and:
   A. ^{99m}Tc DTPA
   B. ^{99m}Tc GH
   C. ^{99m}Tc MAG3
   D. none of the above

18.150 The kidney ROI for a renogram must include the renal:
   A. calyces
   B. cortex
   C. pelvis
   D. A and B
   E. A and C
   F. B and C
   G. A, B, and C

18.151 Film contrast is a property that refers to the:
A. overall blackness of the image
B. differences between the blacks and whites (gray scale)
C. ability to separate two points that lie next to each other
D. amount of distortion of the object being imaged
E. clearness or sharpness of the image

18.152 ^{99m}Tc DTPA aerosol is deposited in the bronchial tree in relation to:
A. air flow rate
B. particle size
C. turbulence
D. all of above

18.153 The presence of LATS (long acting thyroid stimulator) may be an indication of which of the following?
A. thyroiditis
B. Graves disease
C. toxic nodular goiter
D. all of the above
E. A and B only

18.154 Which is the last organ to be visualized during liver/spleen perfusion imaging?
A. kidneys
B. liver
C. heart
D. spleen

18.155 The rate of removal of a tagged colloid from hepatic circulation reflects:
A. the state of blood flow in the liver
B. functional efficiency of parenchymal cells
C. the biological half-life of the radionuclide
D. none of the above

18.156 Indications for SPECT perfusion imaging include all of the following EXCEPT:
A. evaluation of cerebrovascular diseases
B. pituitary microadenoma
C. localization of seizure foci
D. evaluation of head trauma

18.157 When a radiation worker will be exposed to large amounts of radiation are on an infrequent schedule, the monitoring device(s) which would be most useful is(are):
A. thermoluminescent dosimeters (TLD)
B. film badge and ring (TLD) badge
C. pocket dosimeter and TLD
D. A and B

18.158 The basic function of all collimators is to:
A. increase the resolution of the instruments
B. increase the efficiency of the instruments
C. limit scattered radiation
D. limit access of photons to the instrument

18.159 If a technologist consistently runs 14 x 17 inch films so that the replenisher microswitch is activated by 17 inches of film travel instead of 14 inches, the most likely result is:
A. the films will jam
B. the films will be overexposed
C. there will be significant over replenishment
D. an increase in the developer temperature

18.160 Multiple heparinized samples of blood are withdrawn at timed intervals in a plasma determination for the purpose of:
A. reducing the error of random sampling
B. extrapolating the physical decay of the 125 I
C. reducing the radiation load in the patient
D. establishing the rate of diffusion of the albumin from the vascular system

18.161 The purpose of adding hetastarch to the collected blood sample is to:
A. prevent the clotting of the red blood cells
B. prevent the disassociation of the 111In oxine with the leukocytes
C. act as a preservative for the sample
D. bind any indium not labeled to the leukocytes
E. increase the settling rate of the red blood cells

18.162 A radiation beam of 100 mrem/hr is reduced to 25 mrem/hr by an attenuating material. This material is equal to _____ half value layers (HVL).
A. 2
B. 3
C. 4
D. 5
E. none of the above

18.163 Which statement regarding ^{99m}Tc HMPAO is FALSE?
A. it concentrates in metabolically active brain cells
B. uptake is predominately in the white matter
C. it can be used in the evaluation of CVA
D. it crosses the blood brain barrier

18.164 Normal CSF imaging protocols demonstrate the visualization of the radiotracer within the ventricles at:
A. 6 hours
B. 24 hours
C. 48 hours
D. 96 hours
E. none of the above

18.165 32P chromic phosphate is used as radionuclide therapy for the treatment of:
  A. malignant pleural effusions
  B. malignant peritoneal effusions
  C. metastatic bone disease
  D. all of the above
  E. A and B only

18.166 A radionuclide therapy drug used for palliation of bone pain from metastatic disease in patients with breast, lung, or prostate carcinoma is:
  A. ^{99m}Tc MDP
  B. 89Sr chloride
  C. 201Tl Thallous chloride
  D. 32P chromic phosphate

18.167 Before a package that transported a radioactive material can be discarded, you should:
  A. store for a period of ten days
  B. store for a period of ten half-lives
  C. flattened the cardboard to facilitate disposal
  D. deface the radioactive transport label
  E. none of the above

18.168 Which of the following may be considered a drawback encountered in radionuclide bone imaging?
  A. sensitivity to minimal bone changes
  B. nonspecificity of bone abnormalities
  C. uptake in the kidneys and bladder
  D. all of the above

18.169 Which vein of the forearm is most frequently used for venipuncture?
  A. femoral
  B. superior vena cava
  C. median cubital
  D. carotid

18.170 Of the following, the two most important quality assurance measurements of a scintillation camera imaging system are:
  A. focus; astigmatism
  B. energy resolution; counting efficiency
  C. field uniformity; spatial resolution
  D. dead time; resolving time

18.171 The most important factor(s) in determining quality of the tomographic image is(are):
  A. distance from collimator to the patient
  B. number of images acquired
  C. collimator resolution
  D. all of the above
  E. A and C

18.172 Causes for a false negative thallium study would include all of the following EXCEPT:
  A. patient was not exercised adequately
  B. the patient had no complaint of chest pain during the study
  C. planar imaging was performed more than 30 minutes after injection of tracer
  D. there was a global decrease in tracer throughout the myocardium noted in patients with three vessel disease

18.173 Particle size of ^{99m}Tc sulfur colloid preparations are affected by all of the following EXCEPT the:
  A. amount of ^{99m}Tc added to the preparation
  B. amount of gelatin used
  C. heating time
  D. presence of contaminants

18.174 The degree of irradiation resulting from an internally located source of radiation depends on:
  A. the type and energy of the radiation emitted
  B. its physical half-life
  C. its biological half-life
  D. all of the above
  E. A and C only

18.175 A technologist could perform the quality control testing on MAA to include:
  A. instant thin-layer chromatography
  B. particle sizing
  C. limulus amebocyte lysate
  D. all of the above
  E. A and B only

18.176 Which part of the anatomy is least helpful in positioning a patient prior to injection of a radiopharmaceutical for a renal scan?
  A. xiphoid process
  B. iliac crests
  C. umbilicus
  D. costal-chondral margins

18.177 Activity seen in the area of the bowel at 24 hrs on a ^{99m}Tc labeled RBC GI Bleeding study is indicative of:
  A. a positive study
  B. questionable because it may not be at the actual bleeding site
  C. due to breakdown of the tag
  D. all of the above
  E. B and C

18.178 The normal patient undergoing a gastroesophageal reflux examination would demonstrate _____ with an increase of mechanical abdominal pressure.
   A. no reflux
   B. spontaneous reflux
   C. delayed reflux
   D. induced reflux

18.179 In a patient with a gastrointestinal bleeding site, one would expect which of the following changes in blood volumes?
   A. plasma volume will increase; red cell mass will decrease
   B. plasma volume will decrease; red cell mass will increase
   C. plasma volume will increase; red cell mass will increase
   D. plasma volume will decrease; red cell mass will decrease
   E. none of the above

18.180 A LeVeen Shunt imaging procedure using 3 mCi(111 MBq) of ^{99m}Tc MAA is complete when:
   A. the tubing is visualized
   B. the lungs are visualized
   C. the liver is visualized
   D. there is homogeneous activity throughout the abdomen

18.181 Which radiopharmaceutical(s) listed below has been found extremely useful in locating malignant breast tumors?
   A. 210 Tl chloride
   B. 67 Ga citrate
   C. ^{99m}Tc Sestimibi
   D. A and B
   E. A and C
   F. none of the above

18.182 The stannous ion found within a reagent vial may hydrolyze to stannous hydroxide when:
   A. air is introduced
   B. water is present
   C. nitrogen escapes
   D. carbon dioxide is introduced

18.183 The principle radionuclide contaminant of a ^{99m}Tc eluant is:
   A. alumina ion
   B. molybdenum
   C. pyrogens
   D. free pertechnatate

18.184 If a misadministration of a patient dose occurs and is documented on March 3, 1996, the earliest date that those records may be destroyed is:
   A. after March 3, 1999
   B. after March 3, 2001
   C. after March 3, 2003
   D. after March 3, 2006

18.185 Instant thin layer chromatography for water-insoluble radiopharmaceuticals reveals:
   A. percent binding
   B. reduced hydrolyzed
   C. free ^{99m}Tc
   D. radionuclide purity

18.186 In performing a molybdenum 99 ("Moly") break through test, a technologist assays 102 uCi of ^{99}Mo in 950 mCi of ^{99m}Tc pertechnatate. This assay is _____ the allowable limits of _____ uCi ^{99}Mo/mCi ^{99m}Tc for radionuclidic impurities set by the NRC.
   A. outside of; 0.10
   B. outside of; 0.15
   C. within; 0.10
   D. within; 0.15
   E. the same as; 0.10

18.187 A ^{99}Mo / ^{99m}Tc generator is eluted at 2:00 PM for an emergency study and is assayed. The technologist records 47 uCi of ^{99}Mo in 270 mCi of ^{99m}Tc pertechnatate. What should happen next?
   A. the eluate should be tested for the presence of aluminum ion
   B. no testing is necessary for emergency studies performed during the work day; the dose should be drawn for the study
   C. the ^{99}Mo break through is greater than allowable by the NRC and should not be used for patient administration
   D. the radiation safety officer should be notified
   E. B and D

18.188 Good radiation safety measures when handling 32P would include:
   A. use of lead syringe shields
   B. use of lead containers to transport the dose
   C. both A and B
   D. neither A nor B

18.189 Which of the following from a 131I therapy patient would contain the greatest amount of radioiodine?
   A. saliva
   B. urine
   C. feces
   D. sweat

18.190 An Iodine 123 capsule, contained in a glass vial, will result in a _____ when compared to a capsule contained in a plastic vial.
   A. lower assay due to the attenuation of low-level photons
   B. high assay due to contamination
   C. significantly lower assay due to a photoelectric effect

18.191 I-123 has a half-life of 13 hours. A sample of the material has an activity of 5.6 mCi at noon today. What was its activity at noon yesterday? (decay factor = 3.526)
   A. 10 mCi
   B. 15 mCi
   C. 20 mCi
   D. 25 mCi

18.192 The presence of aluminum ions in the ^{99m}Tc eluate is an example of a:
   A. radionuclidic impurity
   B. radiochemical impuriity
   C. colloidal impurity
   D. pyrogenic impurity
   E. chemical impurity

18.193 The radioactive materials precaution sheet which is attached to the chart of the radionuclide therapy patients shall list all of the following EXCEPT:
   A. the predicted date of discharge
   B. the exposure rate at 1 meter from the patient
   C. the radionuclide administered
   D. the administered dose activity

18.194 A 10 uCi dose of 131I was administered for a thyroid uptake study. If the patient's gland weighed 30 grams and their 24 hour uptake was 29%, what was the concentration (uCi/gm), of the 131I deposited in the gland?
   A. 9.7 uCi/gm
   B. 8.7 uCi/gm
   C. .097 uCi/gm
   D. .087 uCi/gm

18.195 In the radionuclide therapy patient's room, exposure rates are measured at which of the following locations?
   A. the patient's bedside
   B. adjacent room
   C. the doorway
   D. all of the above
   E. B and C only

18.196 Urine and excreta from a patient who received a therapeutic dose of 131I in excess of 100 mCi should be:
   A. collected and stored until the radioactivity reaches background levels
   B. collected and stored until the radioactivity is less than 30 mCi
   C. released into the sanitary sewer system as excreted
   D. collected and transported to a burial site with other radioactive waste

18.197 The vasodilatory effects of Persantine (dipyridamole) are reversed by administering:
   A. aminophylline
   B. adenosine
   C. theophylline
   D. dipyridamole

18.198 Which of the following radionuclides is NOT routinely used for lung ventilation studies?
   A. 133Xe
   B. ^{99m}Tc DTPA aerosol
   C. 67Ga
   D. 81mKr

18.199 The majority of radiolabeled particles used for pulmonary perfusion imaging should fall within the range:
   A. below 1 u
   B. 1 to 10 u
   C. 15 to 70 u
   D. 70 to 100 u

18.200 To insure that the radiocolloid therapy agent (32P chromic phosphate) will disperse and cover the wall of the cavity, _____ may be injected into the cavity first and imaged.
   A. 67 Ga citrate
   B. 201 Tl chloride
   C. ^{99m}Tc MDP
   D. ^{99m}Tc sulfur colloid

18.201 Which of the following functions of the liver is utilized in imaging the liver using an "IDA" compound?
   A. bile production and secretion
   B. vitamin and mineral storage
   C. fat metabolism
   D. particulate phagocytosis

18.202 The dose to scan time for ^{99m}Tc sulfur colloid bone marrow imaging is:
   A. immediate
   B. 5 -10 minutes
   C. 60 minutes
   D. 2 hours
   E. 4-6 hours

18.203 Which of the following
radiopharmaceuticals may also be used to
differentiate renal rejection from acute renal failure?
   A. ^{99m}Tc MDP
   B. ^{99m}Tc sulfur colloid
   C. 75Se methioninie
   D. ^{99m}Tc GHA

18.204 When preparing a parenteral injection, it is
essential to keep which of the following areas
sterile?
   A. top of the plunger
   B. needle shaft and tip
   C. exterior of ampule or vial
   D. outside barrel portion of syringe

18.205 The administration of 111In labeled
leukocytes should be accomplished by:
   A. rapid injection through a higher gauge needle
   B. slow injection through a lower gauge needle
   C. slow injection through a plastic tubing
      infusion line
   D. rapid injection using a glass syringe

ANSWERS TO MOCK EXAMINATION

with cross-reference to Chapter and Explanation

18.001	E	1.030		18.034	B	10.050
18.002	B	15.028		18.035	E	11.036
18.003	B	1.024		18.036	A	3.027
18.004	B	6.019		18.037	A	4.016
18.005	A	5.010		18.038	B	5.059
18.006	B	4.054		18.039	C	5.014
18.007	B	3.032		18.040	B	12.012
18.008	A	7.081		18.041	E	11.010
18.009	C	2.029		18.042	C	13.003
18.010	B	8.050		18.043	E	14.020
18.011	E	4.052		18.044	C	15.057
18.012	C	9.041		18.045	D	1.031
18.013	B	1.005		18.046	B	2.023
18.014	D	10.036		18.047	D	6.042
18.015	B	2.026		18.048	E	7.072
18.016	A	11.032		18.049	A	8.044
18.017	F	3.017		18.050	C	9.037
18.018	E	12.021		18.051	A	10.043
18.019	B	4.047		18.052	D	11.018
18.020	G	13.074		18.053	F	12.019
18.021	A	5.060		18.054	C	13.065
18.022	C	5.031		18.055	A	14.026
18.023	B	14.024		18.056	D	15.058
18.024	B	16.026		18.057	C	16.023
18.025	C	17.021		18.058	A	17.015
18.026	A	5.004		18.059	C	1.026
18.027	A	6.014		18.060	A	2.010
18.028	B	1.013		18.061	A	3.024
18.029	C	16.025		18.062	D	4.020
18.030	E	15.034		18.063	B	5.036
18.031	B	7.082		18.064	B	5.043
18.032	B	9.042		18.065	D	5.007
18.033	B	8.037		18.066	B	5.011

18.067	D	6.011		18.105	A	12.015
18.068	A	7.014		18.106	C	5.024
18.069	C	1.008		18.107	B	7.032
18.070	C	2.009		18.108	C	5.026
18.071	D	3.022		18.109	D	16.018
18.072	E	17.020		18.110	A	1.018
18.073	C	4.044		18.111	B	6.033
18.074	C	5.012		18.112	E	11.029
18.075	C	5.015		18.113	F	13.012
18.076	F	6.041		18.114	D	3.018
18.077	B	2.022		18.115	D	17.008
18.078	E	3.021		18.116	B	7.078
18.079	E	17.010		18.117	C	5.006
18.080	B	5.016		18.118	A	4.043
18.081	B	16.024		18.119	D	2.011
18.082	C	15.053		18.120	C	3.014
18.083	D	1.029		18.121	B	17.016
18.084	B	1.022		18.122	A	1.010
18.085	D	5.018		18.123	B	8.048
18.086	C	6.038		18.124	E	9.026
18.087	D	7.021		18.125	E	11.023
18.088	D	1.028		18.126	D	5.025
18.089	E	1.027		18.127	D	12.022
18.090	C	2.018		18.128	A	1.003
18.091	E	8.035		18.129	B	13.057
18.092	C	5.017		18.130	C	14.028
18.093	C	9.028		18.131	D	2.024
18.094	D	1.011		18.132	A	3.031
18.095	D	10.030		18.133	C	16.013
18.096	B	11.033		18.134	B	16.014
18.097	C	5.021		18.135	C	17.007
18.098	E	12.016		18.136	D	10.042
18.099	B	13.053		18.137	A	6.037
18.100	C	13.051		18.138	D	1.004
18.101	D	15.005		18.139	B	3.026
18.102	B	16.005		18.140	B	4.003
18.103	A	17.013		18.141	A	5.005
18.104	A	16.017		18.142	B	5.027

18.143	B	5.038		18.175	E	5.040
18.144	D	5.046		18.176	D	8.023
18.145	A	2.012		18.177	E	13.049
18.146	A	1.006		18.178	A	13.030
18.147	B	7.022		18.179	A	15.023
18.148	D	7.053		18.180	B	13.036
18.149	C	8.034		18.181	E	13.037
18.150	B	8.040		18.182	B	5.048
18.151	B	17.014		18.183	B	5.055
18.152	D	9.039		18.184	D	1.009
18.153	E	10.031		18.185	C	5.058
18.154	B	11.022		18.186	D	5.029
18.155	A	11.012		18.187	C	5.030
18.156	B	12.020		18.188	D	16.031
18.157	C	1.012		18.189	B	16.010
18.158	D	2.006		18.190	A	5.063
18.159	C	17.018		18.191	C	5.013
18.160	D	15.033		18.192	E	5.023
18.161	E	14.025		18.193	A	16.009
18.162	A	1.014		18.194	C	16.015
18.163	B	12.018		18.195	D	16.016
18.164	E	12.009		18.196	C	16.011
18.165	E	16.028		18.197	A	5.035
18.166	B	16.021		18.198	C	5.045
18.167	D	1.021		18.199	C	5.054
18.168	B	6.025		18.200	D	16.030
18.169	C	4.042		18.201	A	5.053
18.170	C	2.004		18.202	C	13.070
18.171	E	3.020		18.203	B	8.042
18.172	B	7.034		18.204	B	4.038
18.173	A	5.064		18.205	B	14.022
18.174	D	16.003				

REFERENCES

Bernier, DR, Christian, PE, & Langan, JK (1994) . *Nuclear Medicine Technology and Techniques* (3rd ed.). St. Louis: Mosby

DuPont Pharma, (1993). *Introduction to Nuclear Cardiology* (3rd ed.). A Professional Education Service of DuPont Pharma Radiopharmaceuticals

Early, PJ & Sodee, DB (1995). *Principles and Practice of Nuclear Medicine* (2nd ed.). St. Louis: Mosby.

Freeman, LM (1986). *Freeman and Johnson's Clinical Radionuclide Imaging* (3rd ed.). Orlando: Grune & Stratton, Inc.

Hole, JW (1994) *Human Anatomy and Physiology.* (6th ed.) Dubuque, Iowa :Wm. C. Brown Company

Mettler, FA & Guiberteau, MJ (1991). *Essentials of Nuclear Medicine Imaging* (3rd ed.). Philadelphia: W.B. Saunders Company.

Palmer, EL, Scott, JA, & Strauss, HW (1992). *Practical Nuclear Medicine.* Philadelphia: W. B. Saunders Company.

Rowell, KR (1992) *Clinical Computers In Nuclear Medicine.* Society of Nuclear Medicine: New York

Saha, GB (1993) *Physics and Radiobiology of Nuclear Medicine.* New York: Springer-Verlag

Sorenson, JA & Phelps, ME (1987) *Phsics in Nuclear Medicine* (2nd ed.). New York: Grune & Stratton

Steeves, A (1992). *Review of Nuclear Medicine Technology.* New York: The Society of Nuclear Medicine

Taylor, A, Jr., & Datz, FL, (1991). *Clinical Practice of Nuclear Medicine.* New York: Churchill Livingstone.

Thomas, CL (1995) *Taber's Cyclopedic Medical Dictionary.* Philadelphia: F.A.Davis Company

Tortora, GJ & Agagnostakos, NP, (1993). *Principles of Anatomy and Physiology.* New York: Harper & Row.